What the experts say about the Fixing Dad programme

'I prescribe Fixing Dad to all my diabetic patients.'

    – Dr Manpinder Sahota (GP)

'Fixing Da   classic. A   le aga nst th
battle to av amputation. A battle to pe   ad
and a battle with general beliefs about type   iabetes.'

    – Roy Taylor, Professor of Metabolic Medicine,
      Newcastle University

'This is a disease that needn't make your life impossible
but you have to make a change in your life that we do
not have a pill for.'

    – Professor Leszek Czupryniak, Chairman EASD

'The reality is that the science has evolved, we now have
a better understanding of the relationship between what
we eat and poor health outcomes. And when armed with
that knowledge we have a moral imperative to act.'

    – Professor Kevin Fenton, Director of Health and
      Wellbeing, Public Health England

'We are used to action as doctors. When something is
going on we get on with it. So it's very frustrating when
politicians and civil servants don't seem to have that
sense of urgency.'

    – Graham MacGregor, Professor of Cardiovascular
      Medicine, Wolfson Institute

Published in the United Kingdom in 2017 by
Short Books, Unit 316, ScreenWorks, 22 Highbury Grove, London N5 2ER

10 9 8 7 6 5 4 3 2 1

A CIP catalogue record for this book is available from the British Library.

ISBN: 978-1-78072-291-7

Recipes copyright © Fixing Dad Ltd
Photographs © Romas Foord

Cover design by Two Associates
Cover image © Levon Biss

Printed at CPI Group (UK) Ltd, Croydon CR0 4YY

The information contained in this book is provided for general purposes only. It is not intended as and should not be relied upon as medical advice. The publisher and authors are not responsible for any specific health needs that may require medical supervision. If you have underlying health problems, or have any doubts about the advice contained in this book, you should contact a qualified medical, dietary, or other appropriate professional.

Caution – before undertaking any of the dietary plans in this book, discuss with your doctor if any of the following apply:

- You have a history of eating disorders
- You are on insulin or a diabetic medication other than metformin – you may need to plan how you reduce your medication to avoid too fast a drop in blood sugar
- You are on blood pressure tablets – you may have to reduce or come off them
- You have moderate or severe retinopathy – you should have an extra screening within six months of reducing or reversing the diabetes
- You have a significant psychiatric disorder
- You are taking warfarin
- You have epilepsy
- You have a significant medical condition

Don't go on the diet outlined in this book if:

- You are under 18
- Your BMI is below 21
- You are pregnant or breastfeeding
- You are recovering from surgery or you are generally frail

FIXING DAD

JEN WHITINGTON

CONTENTS

A message from Anthony Whitington

There's a picture of our dad in 2013, and there's a picture of dad a year later. They are the classic 'before' and 'after' photos. From our first appearances on television in 2014, every press agency wanted these two pictures. Because a picture is worth a thousand words, isn't it?

Well, we grew to dislike those two pictures – and I'll explain why. Unfortunately, if a picture can tell a thousand words, it can also mute a thousand feelings behind a moment, the truth behind a snapshot and where it came from.

'Fat man gets thin' just isn't our story, and we know we wouldn't have got here if it was.

At its heart, *Fixing Dad* is a story about taking personal responsibility for our health and the health of those close to us. But in our two and a half years of Fixing Dad we discovered something else too.

It's quite simple: we have a food industry that pays too little attention to health. And not by coincidence, we have a healthcare system that pays too little attention to food.

As a result, our National Health Service is under huge strain. This is a medical system which does what it says on the tin: it medicates people from one point in time – the point of diagnosis – to an indefinite point on the horizon. Very rarely does it look over its shoulder at what might have caused the problem, and whether we could be brave enough to 'fix' it (or at least attempt to fix it), rather than manage it to death.

My brother Ian and I set out to fix our dad properly in 2013. We also decided to make a film about it, documenting our dad's journey from dire medical prognosis – he was facing an amputation, and his health was in decline – right through to the incredible moment when he was pronounced free of type 2 diabetes.

The process opened our eyes to things we hadn't been prepared for. When it came to health, our beliefs and expectations were tested; we came across methods we had never considered, and might normally have been resistant to trying. Thank God we eventually did try them.

Fixing Dad is the mental, emotional and physical before and after. It's the 'Before Man' who was getting his affairs in order versus the 'After Man' who is in disbelief at his own achievement as he crosses that line, opens that letter from his consultant, and puts his pills in the bin because he no longer needs them.

And on the subject of that 'After Man'… One of the key milestones on dad's road to recovery was when he completed the 100-mile bike ride from London to Surrey. Two years on, we travelled to the Olympic Park to do the same again. Lots of friends asked 'why?' We'd proved our point, they said. We had our medals, so why on earth would we bother?

The truth is that cycling had become much more important for dad than we could possibly have imagined; it was much more than just 'managing his diabetes'. For dad, cycling was the renewed use of his own two feet. It was the wind in the trees, the rain in his face and the sun on his back; it was pedalling along with his wife Marilyn by his side, and spending more time with his grandchildren. It was more time with us – a mixed blessing, I'm sure – but it was, quite literally, the world back at his feet.

Having been buffeted down a catastrophic path of diabetes 'management' for 10 years, he had found a new reality; a new Geoff. And, funnily enough, it was the old Geoff; the one we remembered and missed so much, right in front of us like the cine footage we had compiled for the start of the film we were making about him.

So what will the world make of Geoff's journey? We know there are lots of stubborn mums and dads out there who are facing the same problems Geoff was facing, but for us there are three important things we'd like people to remember.

First, there's nothing special about us. We had the same resources as the next person – an internet connection and blind hope. So anyone can do this.

Secondly, we believe family is the key to unlocking the 'After Man' and the 'After Woman', the real picture that often only our closest families are privy to. We all need to learn how to ask for the support of those closest to us. And if we don't have anyone, then we must ask our doctors for their support; not in 'managing', but in *fixing* our health and finding the support we need. If the doctor isn't supportive, we should consider a change of doctor, just as Geoff had to do.

And finally, we believe the best way of mobilising others to join this cause is simply by raising the question that eluded our family for ten years, but which should matter most to all of us right now: who will I miss when they're gone? And could I help fix them now?

We hope *Fixing Dad* can inspire you on your own journey. Good luck and please stay in touch.

Anthony Whitington
June 2016

Foreword

I have been a part of the Whitington family – Geoff, his second wife Marilyn, and his sons Anthony and Ian – since 1996 when Anthony and I met at university. We celebrated the birth of our first child, Angus, in 1998.

There are several things that struck me immediately about this family, and the three men in particular. The saying that 'The apple never falls far from the tree' is an understatement. Overall they are all remarkably similar. They are all strong-willed and stubborn. They are all prone to volatile over-reactions, miscommunications and rash decisions and one, or a combination, of any of these will crop up every time they are all together.

At times you'd be forgiven for wondering why they choose to spend so much time together at all. But you don't need to look very far to see why. The volcanic outbursts are diffused as quickly as they happen.

There have been conversations over the course of my two decades with them that could tear some families apart at the seams. I have come to the conclusion that this family has no seams. They are a tightly woven fabric of love and loyalty that no one and nothing can unpick. It doesn't occur to them to face anything alone. If one of them is involved then, like it or not, they're all in. I came to this family thinking that I knew what 'family' meant, what it was to be part of one. But this one took me to a whole new understanding.

Ever since I first got to know them, Geoff was the fixer. If anything went wrong, Anthony and Ian would get straight on the phone to him. His phone was on around the clock, he was never further away than 'just down the road' – which covered any distance of up to 100 miles – and he could sort out, rectify or improve anything. Sometimes just by being there. My own dad once said, 'Geoff is the kind of man who turns up and you know everything will be all right.' But in November 2013 his family realised that it was Geoff who needed help. It was time for us all to repay him for the number of times he had been there for us. His sons stepped up to this role wholeheartedly.

This book not only tells that story – of how Anthony and Ian brought their dad back from the brink, helping him reverse his type 2 diabetes – but also outlines a robust and workable plan to show you how you can do the same, either for yourself or for someone close to you. We hope you will be able to use Geoff's story as something of a case study, and an inspiration, for your own health revolution.

We used to joke that everyone should have a 'Geoff' – and now, with the release of the *Fixing Dad* film and this accompanying book, they will.

Jen Whitington
December 2016

PART 1:

THE BEFORE MAN

Behind the statistics

When Geoff stood on the stage at the European Association for the Study of Diabetes (EASD) conference in Croatia, the lectern glaring back at him, a sea of eager and expectant faces turned towards him, he wondered what on earth he was doing there. Geoff Whitington, telecoms engineer of 40 years, whose paper qualifications consisted of an O-Level in woodwork, was standing before an audience of doctors and diabetes specialists. What did he know?

In all those years of running cables Geoff had made a good job of whatever he did – and he wasn't about to make a mess of his job today. He knew his subject inside out: 'Diabetes; the patient's perspective'. He had lived that life for ten years. He knew just how he'd ended up with type 2 diabetes. He knew, too, how much he had wanted to be shot of it. The only way to get his message out was to communicate it with the passion with which he felt it. And there he was, with the people who worked on the front line treating this disease, ready and keen to listen. He cleared his throat.

Geoff's sons, Anthony and Ian, were in the audience. It was with mixed feelings that he glanced at them as he began. In every sense they had put him there – through their love for him, their belief in him... but also, as far as Geoff was concerned, through sheer devilment. They watched him – Anthony from the front row and Ian from behind a camera. Six months ago their dad had sat, exhausted and dejected, on his sofa, his leg resting on the coffee table locked in a protective air boot. The bones in his foot had collapsed making it painful and risky to walk. His other foot was also blighted by diabetic ulcers.

And now here he stood, on his own two feet, keen to tell his story. He had lost several stone in weight, and had gone from taking ten medications to taking only one. Turning things around had proved not to be as complicated as he had once feared. Better still, if *he* could do it, he was fairly certain anyone could.

However familiar you are with the statistics around type 2 diabetes, they never seem to get any less alarming. This is a disease that is covered with such regularity across all media that you might start to feel that it is everywhere. And it is.

Type 2 diabetes is a disease of insulin resistance. The

role of insulin in the body is to bring down blood sugar levels by converting that sugar into energy and driving it to where it is needed in every cell in the body. But a modern diet of sugar and refined carbo-hydrates (which are converted to sugar in the blood), requires more and more insulin to process – and too much insulin causes insulin resistance. Blood sugar levels rise, and the excess insulin can only convert this into fat stores. The fuel is no longer going where it is needed. All of this leads to a build up of dangerous 'visceral' fat on the liver and pancreas, which eventu-ally stops these organs from functioning properly.

The disease is usually, but by no means always, diet related – too many sugary carbs causing a vicious cycle. The good news is that studies now suggest that in most cases type 2 diabetes is preventable and poten-tially reversible by a simple change of lifestyle.

It is important to note that while type 2 diabetes is a disease associated with excess body weight, blood sugar problems can set in without the issue being outwardly obvious. In some unfortunate cases you can become diabetic just from weighing a few pounds more than your particular body type can deal with. Anthony, for instance, had an apparently healthy BMI of 25 and yet he was prediabetic. He, too, had much to gain from changing his diet and lifestyle. The fact is that, for some people, only a minimal amount of excess weight can put you in the prediabetic range. Thereafter it is a small step to full-blown type 2.

Measuring the risk

The only outward indicator that Anthony's blood glucose levels were raised was a slight paunch spilling over the top of his trousers. Abdominal obesity is a pretty clear indicator of internal problems that may be building up and gives some idea of fat distribution in the body. It is a significant sign of an increased risk of any of the health problems that come under the banner of 'metabolic syndrome' – which includes type 2 diabetes and all its associated complications.

There is a simple way to check whether you are in a similar high-risk bracket: measure your waist circumference (the smallest part of your waist, just above your belly button) and divide it by the measurement for your hip circumference (the widest part around your hips and buttocks).

If your reading is above 0.9 for a man, or 0.85 for a woman – especially if your BMI is heading towards, or over, 30 – your health will benefit from undertaking at least part of this programme too.

It is also important here to draw a clear distinction between type 2 and the other main form of diabetes: type 1. This isn't clarified often enough. Around 90% of those with diabetes suffer from type 2. But there are still hundreds of thousands of type 1 diabetics who, rightfully, are often infuriated when a well-meaning Google graduate tells them they might want to cut out sugar and live a healthier lifestyle. Just to be clear – not only are the causes of their condition worlds apart, their treatment and management are very different.

Type 1 diabetes has nothing to do with lifestyle. It happens when the pancreas, for a variety of reasons, fails to produce insulin. The reasons can be complex – especially if you quiz a biochemist about them – but, essentially, it is considered a disease of insulin dependence. As yet there is no cure for type 1 diabetes.

Geoff was suffering from type 2 diabetes, and so references to diabetes in this book relate only to type 2. That said, the potential complications from either form of diabetes are the same: circulatory problems that can result in neuropathy, amputations, heart attacks, strokes, dementia, blindness, organ failure and impotence.

Once diabetes takes hold, the outlook is bleak. The impact on the expected lifespan of a patient, and their quality of life over that time, is significant. One doctor described it to Geoff: 'It's like driving up a mountain track. When you are diagnosed with diabetes, you move from the middle of that track to the outside edge. You're driving with one wheel in the ditch. The risk to your life is now higher.'[1] Current treatment for type 2 is focused on 'management' of the condition. This means increasing levels of medication in an attempt to prevent further systemic damage.

And yet, for many sufferers (Geoff included), a diagnosis of type 2 diabetes does not have sufficient sting. Geoff knew plenty of other people with it; it just meant pills. And in Geoff's case those pills would have lots of company in the cupboard – he was already on medication for raised blood pressure and high cholesterol. He didn't really understand the dangers of the disease or what living with it would mean. He didn't like the thought of having to test his blood sugars every day, but he quickly learned to cope with it as part of his routine. What else could he do? That was how life was now. He resigned himself to an existence in managed decline. He started to make decisions and provisions for his family in the event of his death.

For many years Geoff's family watched on, worried and losing hope of improvement. He had been told

---

[1] Dr Bill Warrilow, GP

by doctors, nurses and podiatrists to change his diet and his lifestyle but neither he, nor his family, knew quite where to start. Sixty years of ingrained habits weren't going to be uprooted overnight. Added to that, Geoff was in no mood for a lifestyle overhaul. His body was failing him and it was zapping his spirit and enthusiasm for everything. It looked unlikely that he would change anything about the situation even if he believed he could. And he didn't. It would take a real scare to jolt us all into action – something that told us that even if Geoff wouldn't change, his circumstances certainly would.

> **Geoff:** I would say to anybody, especially all the diabetics out there: don't give up. Nobody was in a worse condition than me. All you've got to do is get out and do something like this, get on a bike, build yourself up, build your self confidence, and you can get through it.

And that's when his sons decided to formulate a plan to 'fix' their dad.

YOUR ROAD MAP

At the end of each chapter in this book you will find a road map which highlights the key points in Geoff's journey, aimed at giving you the tools and motivation to make your own health revolution. There will be pointers, advice and challenges for you and/or the person you are helping.

There is no pretending that it will be easy, and you may come across resistance – from yourself as well as from others – but hopefully the parallels between Geoff's journey and yours will inspire you to stay the course and keep on the road to better health.

Realising there is a problem

It's not easy watching your rock, your foundations in the world, crumbling slowly in front of you. You can't grab your dad by the collar and shake him, or yell at him that he needs to do something because you can't bear the thought of life without him. Throwing your own emotions at someone

> **Anthony:** We were about to take on the uncomfortable role of parent to our own father...

at such a low ebb in their lives is rarely helpful. This was the position that Geoff's two sons, Anthony and Ian, found themselves in. Geoff had been living with type 2 for nine years. The symptoms were starting to show on the outside. His wife Marilyn was worried about his increasing weight. His ex-mother-in-law, Helen (a retired nurse), noted that 'he wasn't a good colour'. His skin was greyish or very flushed and she was concerned about his heart.

There were other things – he had badly cut his toes whilst trimming his toenails. This wasn't just down to carelessness; rather the nerve damage, or neuropathy, associated with diabetes meant he had little sensation left in his fingers or toes. The poor circulation also meant that any cuts or grazes could easily become infected. He had even burned himself several times in the kitchen and under the car bonnet because he couldn't feel heat through his fingers.

Anthony decided that Geoff needed to break his routine (a vicious cycle of night shifts, after which he would grab sleep when he could and then eat rubbish to cope). Anthony thought that a day out with us and the children would do him good – remind him of all the people who loved him and who he would fight to live for. He came up with the idea of a day at a theme park, and Ian would join us. It had all the makings of being a great day; Geoff, Anthony and Ian were looking forward to it as much as the children were.

There were the predictable ructions in the planning of the day which tend to crop up between these three. Geoff gets frustrated by his sons' inability to organise themselves (why had they not been collecting the vouchers in the newspaper that he had told them to?); they, in turn, get frustrated by his need to control things – and the fact that he associates a day out with having 'a treat' (meaning an overload of cheap junk food).

But it was all innocent enough and, to begin with, the day went well. It was good to see Geoff laughing and enjoying time with his grandchildren. The walking and queuing seemed interminable but everyone had fun. That was until Geoff suddenly stumbled, and just saved himself from falling by grabbing a railing. Anthony helped him up.

Geoff played it down: 'It's my foot. It gave way. It doesn't feel right. I've been walking too much, I suppose.'

It was a long walk back to the car and Geoff was limping badly. Suddenly it hit us all: perhaps this won't be better in the morning.

Geoff was diagnosed by his podiatrist with Charcot's foot – a complication associated with diabetes. It happens when the bones of the foot become weakened by nerve damage. Over years of living with raised blood glucose levels, the tiny blood vessels supplying the nerves – especially in the feet and legs – become damaged. This in turn causes a lack of sensation and weakens the bones, which can then fracture more easily. Because of the lack of sensation, sufferers can continue to walk on a broken foot, exacerbating the condition and causing the joints to collapse. The arch in the foot ends up shaped more like the bottom of a rocking chair. This deformity can fast become a disability and, ultimately, because of the lack of blood flow, can lead to gangrene and then amputation.

Surgery to repair the arch in his foot wasn't an option. Geoff was too heavy for an operation – at over 19 stone, with a BMI of 37, he was considered obese. Either way, the procedure to rebuild the arch wouldn't have been possible with his circulatory problems. There would likely be complications which would almost certainly result in amputation of the foot.

On the surface, Geoff seemed stoical. Enforced rest meant there was little he could do proactively. He felt no need to put up a fight and so spent the next few months recovering at home in his protective air boot, seeing his medication increase. The family once again felt helpless.

Then, one day, the boys realised that the situation had just got a whole lot worse. Now it wasn't just the collapsed foot that was the problem; it was the other one too. There was a sizeable ulcer on his toe. The podiatrist was concerned about the lack of circulation and a conversation about the risk of amputation followed. The whole family felt sick at the prospect. The boys weren't prepared to lose their dad, one piece at a time, to this disease. Ian rang Anthony. Both of them were clearly relieved to talk to each other.

The strong bond between these two brothers comes from years of acute rivalry, of fighting until their noses bled. But it comes also from love and forgiveness. And so, when they have a common goal, they pull together. That night they decided between them on a plan to fix their dad. Little could they have known how successful it would be, and how many people it would inspire; but they were only starting out, and there was a long road ahead.

YOUR ROAD MAP

Deciding to take action

We all adapt to our circumstances surprisingly easily. A shock diagnosis, such as Geoff was given, gradually has less impact as we make room for it and adjust our lives accordingly. When it comes to type 2 diabetes or prediabetes, however, it is important to remember that you don't have to accept it as part of your future. There is a great deal of research and evidence to demonstrate that not only can you halt its progress, in many cases you can reverse it entirely.[1]

---

[1] Professor Roy Taylor, Head of Metabolic Medicine, Newcastle University

Many diabetics – along with their family and friends – are unaware of this and resign themselves to a future they think is inevitable. Their coping mechanism is often to find comfort in old and destructive habits.

Take time to truly consider what is happening – what the future could hold, and what you could do about it, either for yourself or someone close to you. Don't try to solve everything all at once. Focus on the small changes you could make to build new habits. Each time you make a healthier choice you are edging towards a brighter future. More on changing habits later.

The right to intervene

This is an important question, and one that Geoff's sons wrestled with. Geoff is a grown man and a proud one – who were they to bulldoze in and tell him how to live his life? If you are looking to help someone close to you, you will need to address the issue of how best to intervene. The following points should help you navigate this tricky area.

Establishing key areas

While Anthony and Ian felt they had a right to step in and

help their dad, they found that they had to keep the areas in which they helped him very specific. His health, they argued, was their business as, ultimately, it was they who would be partly responsible for caring for him. This Geoff reluctantly accepted. Other aspects of his life remained his business, however, and when they tried to control his working life or home environment, they were firmly batted back in their place.

If you want to help someone who is suffering from type 2 diabetes, you need to be *very clear* about the areas that your help will cover. While you may have your own opinion about what needs to change in their lives, you need to be disciplined about not overstepping any boundaries.

Stay focused on the key aspects of their recovery. After much thought and wrangling, Anthony and Ian decided that their plan would cover three areas of their dad's life:

- Nutrition
- Fitness
- Mind

These points will be the focus of the plan throughout this book. They are tightly interlinked, and when addressing any one of them you need to bear in mind the other two.

The consequences of inaction

If you are in two minds about whether you should intervene at all, considering this point could really help galvanise you. If you do nothing, how will you feel about that? Will you struggle with regret? One thing to be aware of is that the process of supporting someone could end up being as valuable to you as it is to them, and you are likely to improve your relationship and become closer as a result.

Motivation

It had been nine years since Geoff was diagnosed with type 2 diabetes. Popping pills was a way of life; he had come to accept it as an inevitable part of ageing. He was told that he was a sufferer of a progressive but manageable disease and he was gradually seeing the implications of that. He was increasingly losing sensation in his fingertips and toes, and the resulting clumsy accidents (with nail clippers, for example) meant he was no stranger to the GP's surgery. These incidents, he was told, were part of his condition – diabetes could result in circulatory complications. He was now seeing a podiatrist about a toe ulcer as well as a collapsed foot.

The disease was progressing. Geoff was being managed.

Geoff wasn't short of advice on how to slow the progression of the disease, but putting this advice into practice, consistently and sustainably, seemed impossible. Added to this, the advice was often confusing or contradictory. For a man with a below basic level understanding of how his body worked, it tended to have the opposite effect of what was intended. Geoff was finding easy excuses; as far as he was concerned, if the medical professionals themselves were overweight, they clearly weren't following their own advice, so why should he?

The reality was starting to hit home, but not in the way everyone had hoped: Geoff seemed to have resigned himself to living out the rest of his days in ill health. His priority was to get as many shifts in at work as possible to pay off more of the mortgage, should the worst happen. With his health ailing, this relentless workload was tough on his body, playing havoc with his eating habits and metabolism. He spent the bulk of his days off feeling tired and depressed.

There were definitely factors which stopped Geoff from taking control. The first was his attitude to authority. When a doctor told him that he had a condition that would only get progressively worse, he accepted it. These people, in Geoff's view, knew their stuff, and if they pronounced something as fact, he had to accept it as fact: he was on an irreversible downward trajectory.

The second was that Geoff felt a distinct sense of

guilt that he had done this to himself. He had treated his body badly and now it was presenting him with its bill. As far as he was concerned he had little choice but to pay for it. Maybe, in some strange way, trying to sort it out was almost like cheating – he'd asked for it, so he must accept it.

There were other contributing factors that didn't help. For instance, Geoff hated cooking, partly because he felt he had no idea what he was doing. Certainly he had convinced himself that it was more complicated than it is. His wife, Marilyn, was happy to cook for him, and is a good cook, but Geoff preferred to 'spare her the bother', and frequently came home with takeaways. The truth is he probably liked the instant satisfaction to be had from a take-away and to choose his meals rather than have them chosen for him. It all added up and, every day, the diabetes gained ground – as did Geoff's resignation and depression.

The day finally came when the plaster could be removed from his foot. Geoff was relieved. He was to be fitted with an orthopedic shoe and then, presumably, life could go back to normal.

But it wasn't the day of elation Geoff had hoped for. When he sat waiting in the diabetic clinic he was with another man who also had his leg in plaster. Geoff watched as this man was wheeled into the consultation room and watched as he was wheeled out again. To Geoff's horror, the man came out with his trouser leg rolled up above his ankle to reveal a slightly swollen stump where his foot should have been.

This was the moment when Geoff finally woke up to the horrors of this disease. The reality of the suffering, the dependence, the future of rehabilitation, hospitals, perpetual anxiety all hit Geoff like a sledge hammer. He looked down at his leg. Suddenly, the straightforward procedure of removing his plaster seemed fraught with potential complications.

> **Geoff:** I looked at him and I thought, 'That can't be because of diabetes, that can't be...'

What if, when the plaster came off, his foot wasn't better? What if it was worse? What if it was past saving? He felt sick.

'Mr. Whitington please,' came the call.

He lurched in, hoping for the best but fearing the worst. As it turned out, luck smiled back at him that day: he could stand up to this disease one more time.

There is no way of knowing now, but this may have been his final chance.

YOUR ROAD MAP

If you are hoping to help someone close to you then you need to check through several things before you set off on your journey:

Define your motivation

This may be as simple as it was for the Whitingtons: love alone is often enough to power you through the difficult times. You may also be motivated for practical reasons – because you can't cope with that person becoming incapacitated or physically or financially dependent on you. Fear is also a powerful motivator – watching someone's health deteriorate in front of you can be a big contributor to your own stress and unhappiness.

Whatever your reasons for stepping in you need to be very clear about them. You will probably need to communicate your thoughts to the person you wish to help and, if that person is anything like as resistant as Geoff, your reasons will be important in getting him or her on board.

Allocate your time

You need to be honest about the potential demands on

your time. Chances are that you feel every minute is filled to capacity, so it will be tough to find space for additional commitments.

Anthony and Ian both work long hours and the truth is they had to give up a significant amount of their spare time to be there for Geoff. Actively supporting him was crucial, especially at the early stages.

You will need to work out how much time you can give to this project and think about how you will use that time practically. Will you be helping with daily food preparation? Will you supervise or join in any exercise regimes? Can you fit in regular catch-up sessions to review progress?

Build your own support network

We found that there were times when this process could be physically and emotionally draining, and having the wider family around helped Anthony and Ian a great deal. You can embark on this alone but it is tough. Think about who you can turn to for support and encouragement when things get difficult.

Make sure you let them know about your plans before you begin, and get them on side. If nothing else, you'll at least have someone to talk to on the phone when you need a boost.

When helping a diabetic friend or family member,

one way to make it easier to monitor progress, and to empathise, is to overhaul your own lifestyle (though perhaps to a less extreme extent) at the same time. That way you become a support and motivation for each other. You will both benefit in a great many ways.

If you are making a journey of your own

Over the course of filming our documentary and writing this book we have been grateful to receive so many emails from people with similar stories. We've been struck in particular by messages from people who wanted to change things for themselves but had no one to help them through.

For those people all the motivation was there – they were living with the daily realities of declining ill-health and bleak prognoses – but getting information, sticking to a plan and staying positive and focused on their own often proved too tough.

The message here is don't lose heart! In truth, while Geoff had a great deal of support making changes in the beginning, ultimately it was his responsibility to keep enforcing them. You can make significant progress on your own. Think about and cement your motivations, plan how you will use the time you have available to commit to the programme (including food preparation and exercise regimes) and find your own forms of support – even if this is just keeping a journal or video diary. It doesn't matter what form it takes, but you need a progress marker. This will be vital on the difficult days.

The first steps

Geoff was out of plaster, off crutches and definitely in better spirits when he turned up at our house to hear what his sons had in store for him. The way they beamed at him clearly made Geoff rather apprehensive. He had tentatively agreed to work with them to improve his health, but he had, as yet, no idea of the full details.

The boys put it to their dad that they would like to make a documentary about his bid to reverse type 2 diabetes. They wanted him to film himself at home, at work and generally going about his daily life. Geoff agreed, albeit reservedly, and says now that – at the time – he thought he would simply humour them. As far as he was concerned, documentaries required an organisational capability that neither of his sons possessed. For this reason he agreed to do more than he otherwise probably would have.

It started with an interview. This was straight-forward enough. The main goal was to find out, in Geoff's own words, what had led him to his current state. The boys were hunting for the things that revealed the hidden psychology behind his choices. On the surface level there was the drive towards simple gratifications, led by what they referred to as his 'chimp brain'. For Geoff, this meant enjoying food and drink. Enjoyment: that was it; there was no thought of nourishing his body – it was simply a matter of eating what tasted nice. He talked enthu-siastically about his favourite fast food breakfast, the McDonald's Mini Wrap. He talked in wonder about struggling to limit himself to just one serving, sounding like Charlie Bucket telling his family about Mr Wonka's chocolate.

But there were more powerful motivators in Geoff's life, and Anthony and Ian knew it. They needed him to spell them out, to reaffirm them in his own head, in his own words.

'Yes,' he said, without a moment's hesitation. 'Family. Your kids. I don't care what anyone says, your kids come before everything.' This was the launch pad they needed.

Having discussed what it meant to be a dad, they started questioning Geoff about what it was to be a son. Ian asked Geoff about his mum, Elsie. Geoff had never known his dad, and his mum was everything to him. They asked about the last few weeks of her life, and her death, despite being well aware of the answers. There was a point to asking Geoff to go through all the painful details again.

Geoff's mum was a hard worker. She prided herself on this and instilled the same work ethic in her two sons. Geoff never knew her to have taken a day off sick in her entire life. But, like Geoff, she had vices that weren't good for her health – such as smoking.

She died quite suddenly, not long after Geoff and Antonia (Anthony and Ian's mum) divorced. She had been plagued by stomach ulcers but, rather than go to the doctor when she first got symptoms, she kept going, kept working, kept convincing herself that the problem would go away. Finally she was forced to take time off work when the ulcers haemorrhaged. While in hospital, she developed septicaemia and was beyond help. Since her death, Geoff has lived with the regret that more could have been done for her.

It was draining for Geoff to be reminded of the grief of losing his mum and how her health could have been fixed with the right intervention. But now he understood. After several restorative cups of tea and some big hugs, he went home knowing that he would do whatever he had to to prevent his boys feeling the pain he had felt.

YOUR ROAD MAP

Accept there is a problem

First and foremost there *is* a problem. Living with raised blood glucose levels for any amount of time has a dangerous impact on the body on a systemic level. The longer this continues, the more cumulative the damage. Medication is vital in controlling the symptoms of diabetes but it will not deal with the root of the problem.

Obesity can also cause a myriad of other problems. We know that there are many different types of cancer linked to being overweight and, of course, there are the obvious daily bio-mechanical problems that arise, such as issues with joints and movement that, while not life-threatening, certainly impact on quality of life.

Be realistic and honest. What is the current problem? How might it develop? What could be done to improve it? If it is yourself you are trying to fix, the more truthful you can be about the problems, the more effective your solutions are likely to be.

As mentioned earlier, there is increasing evidence to suggest that certain changes and interventions can go a long way towards getting rid of diabetes entirely. Whatever the causes or implications of suffering from type 2 diabetes, it is the body's response to various mechanisms going wrong. Our bodies were designed to be self-healing and there are things we can all do to help that happen.

By accepting that there is a health problem to address, you have taken the first step towards finding a solution.

Talk things through

Getting started is the toughest part. It will involve having some difficult conversations and, if you are the supporter of a diabetic friend or relative, this can be daunting. Find a location to talk which is neutral but comfortable, and have a very clear idea of what you hope to achieve in your discussion. It may take more than one session. Decide whether filming the conversation will be helpful or not – for some people, getting things on record like this can help clarify their thoughts; for others, a camera can make them feel guarded and defensive. You could just record audio or take notes. Consider how a record of these conversations might be a helpful motivator later.

Remember: this can be a painful process. There is no room for judgment, blame or recriminations. In our journey with Fixing Dad we have discovered a common trait in type 2 diabetics – too many carry a sense of shame or embarrassment that they have done this to themselves. Geoff often insisted that it was all his fault. The truth is that there is a myriad of reasons why anyone develops the condition, just as there are numerous causes for blame. The key here is not to point fingers but to empower yourself or a loved one to come out fighting.

Ask questions

What does it feel like to live with diabetes? Are there aspects of it in daily life that this person would love to be freed from? Regularly taking blood readings is pretty grim, as is being at the mercy of medication. Living under a cloud of terrifying statistics can have an oppressive impact on someone's daily life too.

Are there activities or hobbies that you/they once enjoyed but have had to give up due to ill health? How would it feel to be able to go back to them or to start a new activity? What would it feel like to have more energy or see yourself glowing with health?

There are strong links between diabetes and depression[1] and Geoff had clear depressive traits in his behaviour. We will address this point later, but don't be surprised if it feels like you've hit a wall at this early stage. Coming up repeatedly against someone's negativity can be frustrating, but a bit of kindness and understanding can help build a foundation of trust.

---

[1] Professor Arie Nouwen , Psychology, Middlesex University

Find your motivational drivers

Everybody has them. Sometimes they are buried deep, but they are there. With Geoff, facing his bleak prognosis brought his driver to the surface: his love for the people he would be leaving behind. Thankfully these people were as determined as he was to fight for his health and that only served to reinforce his motivation.

Of course, your motivation could be as simple as looking forward to living in a healthier, more mobile version of your body. But make sure you think (or encourage thinking) from the inside out. The clichéd dream of looking great on a beach never works – you'll just end up avoiding the beach! The changes you make need to be real and tangible and make you feel better about this new direction at the end of each and every day.

Employ empathy

By putting their dad back in the position of the bereaved son, Anthony and Ian made him relive the regret and powerlessness he had felt when his mum died. It may seem cruel, but finally Geoff saw how they were feeling too.

If you can get your diabetic friend or relative to understand why you want to embark on this journey with them then you can use the hard times to help build a more positive outcome for you all. It can reinforce their motivation and primary drivers.

If you are making a journey of your own

Taking the time now to reflect on the more unpleasant aspects of your own prognosis may kickstart the momentum you need to take control of your health, one day at a time. Painful as it may be, square up to it. You have it in your power to make a difference to your diabetes and you know that you are sparing your loved ones the hurt of powerlessness and regret.

Then pause for a moment. Be kind to yourself. If you have got this far in the process you are already showing your commitment to better health, and making positive changes to a better future. Keep going forward and make it a reality.

PART 2:

THE PROBLEM

How on earth did we come to this?

As a young man Geoff had a slight and wiry build, so much so that his mum was paranoid that he was underweight and frequently had him checked over by doctors. Elsie was never entirely reassured and made a point of feeding him up whenever she could. Even after he married, Geoff would often stop by his mum's and eat with her before going home to his wife, Antonia, and eating again as a family.

At work, when his colleagues wanted to get down to the pub, Geoff would join them. This was the 1980s. It was a drinking culture. The rule was that you drank a pint of beer every 15 minutes. If it was your round, whether you had finished your drink or not, you went and got the next lot in. This group of men knew themselves proudly as 'The Fat Bastards Brigade'. It was their identity. Money ran through Geoff's fingers faster than the beer ran to his bladder.

To keep up financially, Geoff took evening work in a bar and was away from home longer. He felt guilty about the time away from his kids, and his first marriage fell apart. When he remarried, he tried to embark upon more positive habits. But rather than live more healthily, and treat his body better, he simply kept his vices to himself. The let-downs and monotony of his daily life perpetuated the cycle – drinking, spending, inactivity and self-denial.

Geoff spent most of his time on the road for work and saw fast food as the most economical and realistic option for him. He had no means of refrigerating a packed lunch and no interest in preparing one. He had a job to do that required maximum efficiency. Food had to happen quickly.

> **Geoff:** Living my life as I did, with all that weight and all the drink and everything else… it wasn't going to do any good, was it? You think it's just diet, you think it's just fat, you think it's just putting on weight, but it affects your whole being.

A compulsory 'Over 40s Health Check' for work was about to reveal the extent of his problems. It hadn't helped that his motorbike had broken down on the road and he'd had to push it all the way to the medical centre. It also didn't help that Geoff suffered from an extreme case of what professionals call 'white coat syndrome' – a deep-seated discomfort with hospitals that can manifest itself in, among other things, a rise in blood pressure.

For most patients adversely affected by a hospital environment, multiple blood pressure checks over the duration of their visit, as they relax over time, usually iron out the early, anomalous results. Geoff doesn't remember what that first reading was. He remembers the nurse blanching as she read it, resolving to take it again when he'd calmed down. He remembers mutterings along the lines of 'I'm not sure that's possible'. But the second and third readings weren't all that much better. He remembers that he had a cholesterol reading of 15 and was told that was high, but he admits that at that stage he had no idea of the potential consequences of these results. Had he not been told later that he had three months to get these readings to safe levels or he would lose his job, he might not have done anything at all.

And so it began – Geoff's numerous, and ultimately failed, dieting attempts. He was put on medication for his blood pressure and cholesterol – so he was slightly less of a health time-bomb than on the day of his medical – but he still needed to lose weight. Geoff's story with dieting is probably not that different from the stories of other overweight people. He leapt from one thing to another. He tried cutting right down and then almost starving himself (if less food would get him to the weight he wished to be, then no food would get him there faster and then he could get back to normal). He would eat oranges, lots of oranges, nothing but oranges. But he thought that whatever weight he lost gave him room for manoeuvre – and that meant blowouts. It is only really now, all these years later, that Geoff has been able to be honest about how alarming his eating habits became in those days.

Geoff's dieting attempts were not just unrealistic, but went as far as to compound failure in his head: 'It has never worked before, why should it work this time?'

Well, he is living proof that it can be done. We eventually found a diet that worked for Geoff and which, crucially, fulfilled his criteria of fast results. It has a special place in this book, not only for its effectiveness against type 2 diabetes and prediabetes, but also because of the groundbreaking man who inspired it.

As Anthony and Ian sat together, formulating their plan for Geoff, they knew nothing of these beacons of hope. But Geoff had committed, in theory, to their project and his sons believed that their dad could do anything. That belief was all they really needed.

YOUR ROAD MAP

Increasingly we are all leading busier and more exhausting lives and we often forget to look up at where we are going. Before you know it you can be a long way down a path you didn't intend to take. Remember that you can change it. Make time for the things that matter. Your well-being is paramount.

The role of wider family and friends

We like to think that those around us will be supportive of our efforts to lose weight but it can sometimes cause friction. People can take our refusal of a drink on a night out, or of a slice of cake, as a judgment of their behaviour, and can become defensive. Try responding differently: rather than saying, 'No thanks; I'm on a diet,' try explaining how you are trying to take back control of your health, and even that you might need their help along the way. People are far less likely to push if they are invested in your journey.

The other aspect to consider is that your changed behaviour will bring about a sort of identity shift and will alter other people's understanding of who you are as a person. Consciously or not, we tend to place our nearest and dearest in neat little boxes. Our family did it with

Geoff; and we all constantly do the same with people we know. *'I'll get a packet of shortbread for him because he loves that'* is a stance that, however well-meaning, will make things difficult for someone on a diet. *'She'll want to stop and get cigarettes so I'll ask her to fill the car up with petrol while she's out'* is an unhelpful suggestion for someone who wants to quit smoking. *'She would never come and watch that film with me because she hates chick flicks'* may be fair enough, but that person could benefit from spending some time with a friend, whatever the activity.

Nobody means it destructively; we do it simply because it is comforting to stick with the familiar, and to think how well we know someone we love. In the Whitington family, we all had trouble adapting to the new, upgraded, disciplined and more self-respecting Geoff, even though we had instigated the changes ourselves.

A note on moderation

If there is one phrase we have heard more than any other over the course of this project it is that 'everything is fine in moderation'. The problem with this is that moderation is a subjective term. One person's view of moderation is not the same as another's. Geoff was visiting drive thrus seven times a day at one point; so calling in just once a day was his idea of abstinence – but a burger a day is a recipe for weight gain, so this interpretation of moderation was not getting him anywhere. Be honest about where you or your loved one want to get to and double check that the decisions you make about food are moving you forward.

Habit breaking

Habits fast become the unthinking auto-pilot of our everyday lives. If we eat the same foods, in the same places, from the same takeaways, and permit ourselves the same snacks, the thought of changing our routine can seem unbearable. Remember that unless you make a change, *nothing* will change. A simple change of behaviour – such as preparing your own meals – will make a huge difference (more guidance on this later).

With Geoff it was about showing him how quickly small changes added up to something big: cut out the sugar/sweeteners in your tea; park further away from your destination and leave later so you have to walk fast; pace the floor when you're on the phone; have a glass of water instead of a snack... It all seems small and insignificant but you are reprogramming your brain and resetting your body.

Speak to your GP

By now you, as supporter, have committed to a project to help someone you care about. Hopefully you have their commitment too. Remember that this is a serious under-taking and make sure you have the support of the GP overseeing this person's care. Not all doctors are receptive (Geoff's original GP was less than enthusiastic). If they are not, you need to know why. Some GPs are simply pessimistic about their ability to support a patient through the process. On the other hand, their doubts could be due to genuine concerns about medication or potential dangers to health. It is important to discuss your plans with your doctor and to work out a safe way forward. There will usually be options for you.

Identifying the sweet spot

When we started the process of fixing Geoff's health, we assumed that the reasons for developing type 2 diabetes rested firmly with the individual. This picture becomes much more complicated, however, when you look at why so many people have become heavier over the years.

Our research into how best to fix Geoff's health led us to speaking to some serious academics who make it their business to know as many sides of this issue as they can.

Professor Susan Jebb, a government adviser on obesity, put it the most diplomatically when she said, 'You either have to say that there has been a national collapse in willpower or you say "Wait a minute, the world has changed".' She says that, for years, the business model in the food industry has been based on selling us products which are higher and higher in calories and that this business model is undermining our health.

Jebb is a pragmatic woman. To her, it seems reasonable to expect that the food industry could use its understanding, and its ingenuity, to supply us with food that is supportive of our health, rather than detrimental to it.

The dilemma for the food manufacturer or supermarket is a big one: if you make efforts to substantially reduce the levels of sugar, salt or saturated fats in foods you run the risk of altering flavours too much and losing your customers. Sugar, salt and saturated fats make up the holy trinity of palatability in processed foods; if you reduce one you must increase the others to compensate.

This is, essentially, how we ended up in this dire situation in the first place.

In the 1970s and 1980s there was great war on fat in food due largely to studies – now discredited – into the role of body fat and its supposed link to coronary heart disease. The industry responded by massively reducing the fat in its products. This seemed all well and good, except for the fact that nothing tasted quite as good when it was low fat. So they rectified this by adding more sugar or more salt. The problem, on a production level, was solved: the fat content was lower and we, the consumers, were delighted that our favourite foods were, according to the science of the time, now better for us.

The science, however, is now yelling in our faces. These higher sugar foods that we have lived on for years and grown accustomed to – even dependent upon in our cravings for them – are massive drivers of insulin. Remember this is a fat storing hormone. When we eat these things, even in 'moderate' amounts, we are habitually forcing our bodies to produce more and more insulin. This applies whether you are type 2 diabetic or not. Consistently eating these foods will put a cumulative strain on your body that it may or may not be able to cope with in the long term.

While the figures relating to the number of diagnosed type 2 diabetics across the world are alarming, the number who are undiagnosed or prediabetic and unaware of their condition is terrifying. This is true both in terms of the cost to our health services, but also in terms of what it will do to families who will have to help deal with the resultant health complications, and who will have to watch loved ones gradually dying in front of them.

Real, hard solutions on a macro level seem a long way off. So many of the experts we spoke to are taking increasingly activist stances – from Dr Aseem Malhotra, cardiologist and founder member of Action on Sugar, who talks openly of the 'greed and excesses of the food industry', to the group's chairman, Graham McGregor, Professor of Cardiovascular Medicine at the Wolfson Institute, voicing his desperate frustration at the lack of government action on this issue.

Both men campaign endlessly for solutions to the obesity epidemic and a big part of their work involves putting pressure on the government to reinstate regulatory measures that will protect the public. Professor McGregor filled us in on the current situation.

Under the previous Labour government we had the Food Standards Agency. They had powers to regulate our food industry in the UK, including enforcing guideline levels of salt, fat and sugar in our food. The playing field was level in the respect that all manufacturers and producers were abiding by the same rules.

With the change of government, Andrew Lansley disbanded the Food Standards Agency in favour of the 'Responsibility Deal'. This was a voluntary code of conduct for the industry, so its members could choose to sign up to its guidelines or not. Predictably, most of them did not. When profit is at stake, volunteers for such measures are thin on the ground. Lansley's decision to make these changes was subject to fierce debate and criticism, but, either way, these changes were made.

In the end, the Responsibility Deal was a failure. Professor McGregor, like many others, sees increased government regulation as central to finding a solution. This is not a man with a bee in his bonnet. He has attended autopsies on children as young as four years old with early stage atheroma (where their arteries are blocked or swollen by fatty deposits). Poor diet is a big contributor and it is affecting more people, and doing so at an earlier stage in their lives, than ever before.

I witnessed a Twitter debate where one user described the 'obsession with sugar' as 'a neurotic middle class problem'. The reference to social class was a means of trivialising the issue as one that only those with little to worry about might get hysterical over. The truth is that this disease is indiscriminate. It affects people from all walks of life, all backgrounds, and all levels of education. Doctors like Dr Malhotra and Professor McGregor know this to be the case. They are the ones performing life-saving operations, telling relatives that there is nothing more they can do, having to go home and live with it and still go into work the next day and do it all again.

So, do we still believe that the responsibility for this disease lies with the individual sufferers or do we share Professor McGregor's opinion that it lies as much if not more with the food industry? Or is it that the government has seriously let us down? After all, how many people knew that government nutritional guidelines had, for years, been funded by industry and had nothing to do with World Health Organisation recommendations?

It appears that this health epidemic is a result of all of these factors combined: a dangerous cocktail of government inaction, consumer manipulation by the food industry, and our own behaviours.

Take the sweets at the check-out, for example, and the placing of certain brands at eye level or on the endcaps of aisles in the supermarkets. Aggressively targeted advertising campaigns bombard us so continually that their messages play on us subliminally all through our day. At the same time, manufacturers respond to market demand. If consumers prefer to buy five donuts for £1 instead of a bag of spinach, supermarkets will stock their stores accordingly. Our senses and decision-making processes are then shaped by the overly accessible, poor quality, nutritionally invalid food that makes up the bulk of our immediate view as we shop. The problem is self-perpetuating.

Any one individual with type 2 can well argue that he or she is a victim of industry or market forces but, as a collection of individuals, we have the ability – and responsibility – to break the cycle. If we stop demanding these foods, they will not be so aggressively marketed and fewer people, in turn, will be manipulated into buying them.

By changing your food choices every time you shop you are shaping the market forces and the operating guidelines and objectives of these manufacturers. You are making that decision for them three times a day, with every meal you eat or feed to your family.

YOUR ROAD MAP

Know what you eat

It is at the discretion of food manufacturers to decide what they put in their food. They know that marketing something as 'healthy', 'natural' or 'low fat' fits with what most of their customers are looking for. It is only when you look very closely at labels that you realise that all those terms are subjective and not measured according to any universal standard. Public Health England have recommended that the government bring food labelling into line with World Health Organisation guidelines, particularly in relation to sugar and salt, but as yet this hasn't happened. RDIs (Recommended Daily Intakes) currently tally with the Department of Health's recommendations but these are far in excess of the amounts the WHO deems safe.

Moves are in place to change this but, as it stands, there is no means of enforcing compliance from companies. As consumers, we really have only one defence against this: to try as much as possible to use foods in our kitchens that have no ingredients lists – that is, food that is a single whole ingredient: a fresh chop, eggs, spinach, nuts, olive oil. This isn't always possible, of course, but aim to cook from scratch as much as you can. The guidance in this book will help you along the way.

Preservatives

To help keep things fresher for longer companies need to use preservatives. These can be as basic as a load of salt (as in commercially produced bread that has roughly eight times the salt content of a homemade loaf), but there are also more complex varieties. Sadly they won't preserve *you* like some magical elixir of youth, but they will keep doing the job that they are designed to do right the way through your body, a process which kills bacteria. This property of preservatives is good for food shelf-life but it is fairly disastrous for your intestinal tract. You have millions upon millions of valuable and necessary bacteria in your gut that are vital to sustaining your overall health. As the preservatives pass through, they wipe them out.

The other thing that helps to keep food shelf-stable (and make it quicker to cook up at home) is the deliberate removal of fibre. Our overall fibre intake today is a fraction of what it used to be and fibre is essential for helping these important bacteria do their job.

Processed food

Food manufacturers don't make food in the same the way you would in your kitchen, whatever their ad campaigns tell you. Their production is carried out on an industrial scale – and has to be so. This results in industrial levels of potential bacteria and consequent clean-up materials (read the percentage ammonia content on a product containing minced meat of any sort). This is not about generating hysteria, but simply that, if you want to make sure that you know what you're eating, it is best if you prepare it yourself.

I provide plenty of easy, nutritious meal options later in this book to give you a no-nonsense guide to sticking to things that are good for you.

PART 3:

THE FIX

Nutrition

Right. To action! We now need to look at the three key areas Anthony and Ian focused on with their dad: nutrition, fitness and mind.

Getting the diet right

There are diets circulating in every bookshop, newspaper or internet forum. Chances are that, with perseverance, any one of them may help you, or your diabetic charge, to lose some weight. The problem is that, for a diabetic, the *type* of food they eat is even more important than the amount of it – certain foods pose a bigger problem than others. As we have seen, the misguided demonisation of fat in the 1970s and 80s led to a prevalence of low-fat foods and eating plans. Unfortunately, those who were put on low-fat diets

– including diabetics – were guided towards regimes that were high in carbohydrates. The rationale was that carbs would fill you up fast and give you energy to power you through your low-calorie day. There are some people for whom carb-loading can be useful – such as serious endurance athletes – but for most of us it is detrimental, and a key cause of weight gain.

Thankfully, these days, recommended diets for type 2 diabetics increasingly involve low-carb guidelines, often in conjunction with a higher fat quotient. To understand why this shift in opinion is taking place, we need to understand how carbohydrates function in our bodies and how they affect diabetic bodies in particular.

Dr Warrilow, Geoff's new, forward-thinking GP, had already explained to us that years of excessive carbohydrate consumption (in the form of sugary, starchy foods and alcohol) had caused Geoff's system to become flooded with insulin, putting strain on his pancreas and causing the cells in his body to become insulin-resistant. Dr Malhotra told us more. He explained that carbohydrates drive insulin in our bodies more than fats or proteins. This is because carbs – especially refined carbs – are turned into sugar in our bodies and insulin is released to convert those sugars into energy.

So there you have it: too many refined carbohydrates,

leading to too much sugar, leads to too much insulin and eventually insulin resistance. Soon those blood sugar levels are rising, and the body is over-producing insulin, piling extra calories into fat stores rather than converting them to energy. Hence Dr Malhotra, who has been tireless in getting this message out to the people who need to hear it (whether they be sufferers, their families, doctors, politicians or the media), summarises type 2 diabetes as 'a disease of carbohydrate intolerance; the body's inability to metabolise carbs'.

Changing Geoff's diet

Even with this advice now circulating widely in relevant circles, not everyone seemed to agree on it, so with Geoff we had to forge our own path and devise a plan that worked for him.

We knew Geoff's diet should be low in carbohydrates so we had a good starting point. We also kept it pretty low in saturated fat, just to be sure! (Increasingly, research shows that actually we need not have worried so much about this. These days Geoff is still on a low carbohydrate diet but he makes up much of his calorie intake from fat. It keeps him full for longer and helps him to stay off the carbs.) The new way of eating meant that, on a simple level, Geoff's plate went from being mostly beige to mostly green.

To keep things simple we kept the guidelines to proteins, healthy fats and surface-growing vegetables i.e. no root veg (which meant no potatoes but lots of courgettes, lettuce, cabbage, runner beans and so on). Bread was off the menu entirely, much to the disappointment of the man who could almost consume a baguette whole.

The obvious culprit that also had to be completely eliminated was sugar.

We got mean. We didn't just strip sugar from his diet, we stripped out all sugar substitutes too – including artificial sweeteners – both because we needed to reduce his craving for sweet things and because these substitutes are thought to have a disastrous effects on gut bacteria.

Alcohol, too, was completely off the menu for two months.

For anyone who is worried by the sound of this, remember: low carb is not the same as no carb. Geoff was still getting good carbohydrates from fresh vegetables – it was just anything

> **Geoff:** You can buy it, but I'm not gonna eat it.
>
> **Ian:** Have you ever tried it?
>
> **Geoff:** No I'm not gonna try it. I will not eat that... thing.

that was going to force high spikes in insulin that was out. This even meant limiting fruit – especially the tropical varieties, like the humble banana – which in turn meant that it was even more crucial that he got the required nutrients and fibre from vegetables. He learned to enjoy nuts and he had to get over his issues with fish (we had to make some compromises but he ditched the battered variety). He ate a wider variety of meat and fish, and gradually he started to feel not just better but astoundingly well.

Getting confident in the kitchen

While some of the rules over what Geoff could and couldn't eat may look complicated, the key tenets were actually quite simple. What was more complicated however, was getting *him* to take control over what went into his meals. And that meant getting him cooking – something well outside Geoff's comfort zone. Anthony and Ian took charge, but Marilyn supported wherever she could. It was a learning process for everyone, including the boys!

When we talked (or argued) with Geoff about his role in the kitchen, we discovered that most of what he 'hated' about cooking was his own ignorance as to how to go about it. Our challenge was to devise a plan for someone who had no idea about shopping, chopping, cooking and washing up. He wouldn't want to bother with food that he had to watch for hours on a hob and that involved lengthy prep. He didn't want 'fancy' ingredients so they all had to be pretty run-of-the-mill, buy-it-in-the-supermarket-type foods; he wasn't going to be visiting any specialist grocers or health food stores. Geoff doesn't have a food processor and his knife skills aren't great because of his numb fingers, so we knew our estimations of prep times couldn't be over-ambitious.

Primarily, we wanted to show him that cooking is not complicated, time consuming or expensive, and that you can just toss a few ingredients into a pan and then onto a plate. Cooking in one vessel (whether pot, dish or wok) minimises washing up, and using the oven rather than the hob means less standing around guarding pans. If you want cuts of meat to cook faster you can bash them flat with a rolling pin. Otherwise fish or eggs can be a decent substitute as they cook quickly. Veg, as always, is a winner, because its high fibre content helps to fill you up.

Geoff wanted to know exactly what he would be eating each week and wanted a detailed shopping list – so we compiled that too. You can find the successful shopping lists we hit upon in the final section of this book. He also needed some packed lunch options, including foods that could survive out of the fridge for a bit longer in case he was out on the road.

A popular misconception about diabetics

Many people said to us that surely Geoff 'needed' sugar as a diabetic because his body couldn't produce it naturally – but this viewpoint was simply a confusion of the mechanics of type 1 and type 2 diabetes, probably stemming from the fact that type 1 diabetics have difficulty producing *insulin* and so can't convert blood glucose into energy. In each disease, the sufferer can experience what is known as a 'hypo' if their blood glucose levels do drop too low to provide sufficient energy for the body. Type 2 diabetics are at risk of this on certain medications – and as Geoff lost weight and his blood sugar levels began to regulate his medication could become too high for what his body now needed. This is one of the reasons why medical supervision and diligent monitoring is so important when undertaking this sort of dietary regime.

Discovering the 8-week plan

One of our key strokes of luck came when we found

out about a groundbreaking study which, at the time, was just a gleaming gem of promise that lay hidden to most. Up in Newcastle, Professor Roy Taylor, Head of Metabolic Medicine, and his team of researchers had developed a programme designed to halt and even reverse type 2 diabetes. Professor Taylor kindly found the time to talk to us about how it worked.

The premise of Professor Taylor's successful programme has one critical component: all of his patients are put on an extremely low-calorie diet. They are restricted to eating around 800 calories a day for six to eight weeks. You may have heard about the regime after it made headlines in 2016, largely thanks to Dr Michael Mosley's *8-Week Blood Sugar Diet*, which is based on Prof Taylor's research; and you may have thought it sounded quite extreme. Geoff is now one of the success stories, and this book is designed to demonstrate how achievable it is when done correctly.

Prof Taylor's advice certainly doesn't end at the short-term 800-calorie rule. There are important points and precautions to take on board and we had to keep these at the forefront of our thinking. Most importantly, any eating plan we devised for Geoff had to be balanced and nutritious and contain sufficient healthy fats for his daily energy needs. But with this new plan at our disposal we reworked Geoff's low-carb diet, decreasing the calories further to match the Newcastle Diet guidelines, while being careful to ensure it was appropriate and nutritious.

Could it work?

When he started out on his initial 8-week regime, Geoff had his own interpretation of cutting calories: he figured he'd have to eat some veg and some unbattered meat or fish but, having prepared it all, he would then upend a jar of pre-prepared sauce on it. When you are used to such sauces, neat vegetables can feel a bit tedious.

Clearly these sauces, which are loaded with salt, sugar and preservatives, had to go.

The edict to cook everything in one pot helped in this regard – it allowed all the flavours to be layered together without leaving Geoff with a pile of unappetising steamed veg on the side.

From now on, Geoff had to know exactly what he was putting into his food. Encouraging him to inject natural but interesting flavours was all part of a plan to reset his taste buds and show him that he was going to feel and look better, inside and out.

Anthony and I did a test run of the short-term low-cal, low-carb diet ourselves to see how we functioned. Could we keep up with the kids, jobs, exercising, driving and socialising on an 800-calorie day? Could we fit in providing extra food for the children who needed significantly more filling up? Was it likely to add much to our food bill? Would our draining board look like a cityscape with its towers of pans?

I am generally exhausted from the daily routine by 9pm, so meals need to happen quickly and with minimal washing up – and we were pleased to find that our proposed new diet didn't throw in a load of extra timing and culinary challenges. Yes, Geoff would be slower – he, after all, wasn't used to any sort of cooking (while our kitchen at home can be a well-oiled machine, given that we already cook daily for six) – but we felt there were no curveballs that arose from the new routine.

We also found within a fairly short time that the more natural the flavours we ate, the less we craved the artificial foods that we had eaten in the past. If anything, they actually became pretty repellent. It was as though eating only natural flavours switched on an awareness of artificial ones – something that would be a real benefit for Geoff. If we could just get him to stick with it, not only would he stop craving those things, he would actively avoid them. Ideally, his taste buds would change for good so that after he had completed the 8-week 800-calorie phase and moved on to a low-carb maintenance model, he would retain this appetite for healthier food.

In the end, Anthony and I didn't find that we struggled too much on lower calories. We had to recalibrate our approach to hunger a little (such as having a glass of water or a tea when a mild hunger pang might otherwise have fooled us into snacking), but we got through it without feeling any real discontent.

Making progress

To start with, Geoff found the regime difficult. Going without his beloved sugar was like a form of cold turkey for him. He got irritable. He felt tired. His mood dived. And things continued this way for a week. But then... he emerged on the other side.

The difficulties in that first week began to be offset by the positive progress he made: in three days he lost five pounds. We were well aware that initial weight loss on a diet is often water so we tried not to get too excited. Plus, we didn't want quick weight loss to be part of a yo-yo cycle. But it looked to be nothing of the sort. Geoff was so delighted to see the weight coming off that it spurred him on and sharpened his resolve. Suddenly it seemed he was quite indifferent to his previous diet staples.

He was a bit alarmed by the amount of veg he had to eat but he had orders to follow. We had tried to counter his objection to vegetables by adding variety: if one type of veg wasn't a favourite, he could mix it up with others or try a different way of preparing it. We got past a dislike of the taste and texture of aubergines by using them as the base in an aubergine 'pizza' – thinly sliced, grilled, and topped with tomatoes, garlic, olives and cheese.

Sure enough, after just a few weeks he started to glow. He looked visibly younger and was much more energetic and enthusiastic about everything. He got more proficient in the kitchen and, during those first eight weeks, his taste buds definitely changed. The pressure he was taking off his system meant that, even in the reduced-calorie phase, he didn't find himself especially hungry. Before long this regime became self-rewarding and new habits were forged. Rather than hiding in his old comfort zone of enforced denial about what he was eating, he started separating the good from the bad, admitting that certain foods just weren't doing him any favours.

The 8-week low-calorie diet was a revelation and one that truly transformed Geoff's health. He subsequently went on to a low-carb maintenance plan that adhered to the same guidelines regarding which foods to eat (fresh meat with fat, oily fish, surface-growing veg), but included more healthy fats and wasn't restricted to calorie counting.

It really was that simple – and effective.

YOUR ROAD MAP

The term 'diet' was heavily loaded for Geoff, as it is for countless people. For many it becomes a kind of short-hand word for all the feelings associated with years of hopping from one regime to another; a spiral of denial, exclusion, hunger, discomfort, disappointment and failure. These elements need to be removed from the equation, and the easy approach to healthy eating outlined in the final section of this book should help you with this. Remember: this is less about 'diet' and more about moving towards a long-term, sustainable approach.

The 8-week low-calorie phase

To follow the plan that worked for reversing Geoff's diabetes, you will need to embark on a short-term diet cutting right back on refined carbohydrates and reducing your calorie intake to approximately 800 per day – *N.B. this low-calorie phase is for six to eight weeks only*. You need to ensure you are still getting the all-round nutrition your body needs, which means a balance of good ingredients in your meals. The list below provides an outline of what foods are in or out, and the itemised shopping lists in the final section of this book will give you a hassle-free guide to what to put in your supermarket trolley.

Prof Taylor's research is based on rapid weight loss stripping visceral fat from around the organs and correcting the body's mechanisms for regulating blood sugar and insulin. People get worried about so-called 'crash dieting', but there is strong evidence out there now disproving the idea that the faster you lose weight, the faster you put it back on. You certainly shouldn't continue restricting your calories in the long term (as I have said, the 800-calorie-a-day diet is for just six to eight weeks). Beyond that period, as part of an ongoing maintenance plan (see p.95) you do need to stick to a low-carb regime, but you can stop counting calories and introduce more healthy fats. Armed with this, there is no reason why you, or your diabetic friend/relative, should pile the weight back on simply because you have lost it quickly. In fact, for Geoff, getting down to a new, low weight fast was hugely motivating and made him feel more in control of what he was eating.

What foods to eat

- Foods low in refined carbohydrates

- Healthy fats and some protein
- Surface-growing vegetables only, i.e. no root veg
  (which means no potatoes, but lots of greens, such
  as courgettes, lettuce, cabbage, runner beans etc)
- No bread, rice or pasta
- And, of course, no sugar

Know your macros

Fat, protein and carbohydrates are referred to as macro-nutrients – and we need them in our bodies – but they are not all created equal.

Fat

Fat is not only satiating – helping us to stave off hunger – it is also essential for our bodies. The good news for type 2 diabetics is that it won't affect insulin levels either. Even when on a lower-calorie diet, it's very important that a good proportion of calories comes from fat.

We put the emphasis in Geoff's diet on healthy natural fats – as found in nuts, avocados and oily fish. For this reason, we included butter, coconut oil and olive oil but stayed clear of artificial fats such as margarines and vege-table oils.

Protein

All of us need protein, and Geoff's muscles particularly needed it as his exercise programme (see next chapter) began to pick up pace. If you are not a vegetarian you can get most of your protein from animal-based sources such as meat, fish and eggs. Legumes and pulses are good plant-based sources of protein but they are also fairly high in carbohydrates, so you have to be a bit careful about how you use them.

Carbohydrates

This is not a dirty word, even for type 2 diabetics – again, it is about the quality of those carbs. The big, green vegetables that Geoff originally had such an issue with provide high quality carbohydrates and a load of fibre and micronutrients too.

Get shopping and get cooking

At this instruction, as we've seen, Geoff recoiled in horror and almost abandoned the project. But it's not complicated and it's not scary. It doesn't require tons of planning; you don't need expensive ingredients, equipment or a shelf full of recipe books, nor will it take up all of your time. Later in the book there are examples of weekly shopping lists and everyday recipes that worked for Geoff and will really simplify things for you. These recipes are also designed to require minimal equipment to save clear-up time.

When you're shopping, stick to ingredients that do not need to display an ingredient list – in other words, use whole foods as much as possible. That way you know nothing has been added to your meals that you'd be better off without. Item for item these whole ingredients may seem more expensive than a ready meal but there are often leftovers that can go in a packed lunch the next day. Anything you don't use one week can also be frozen for another week to save time and money. There are plenty of ways to use simple, whole ingredients in efficient and inexpensive ways, so don't be afraid to experiment with what you have.

Your new way of eating can be made less painful by not having pockets of temptation in the house. It is hard enough steering a clear path through these ever-present and aggressively marketed products out in the wider world, but home should be a sanctuary from this battle with willpower. For the most part, our food choices are not the measured and considered decisions that we like to kid ourselves they are. Generally they are pretty impulsive and based on the food in our immediate environment. So keep temptation out of reach.

If you or your diabetic charge are not the main shopper

in the house, make sure you get the person who does the shopping on board with your plans. They may hold the keys to success or failure based on how they stock the kitchen.

Keep a diary

One well-understood standard of dieting support is accountability. This is because it is tied in with conscious eating, reinforcement of new habits and shared success. It is why members of dieting support groups have more successful outcomes than those going it alone.

We made Geoff document, and later measure, exactly what he was eating and when.

It is important that you, or the person you are helping, has a constant and accurate account of what they are eating. While this sounds like a tremendous hassle, it needn't be. It can be as simple as a written food diary or photo journal, or something as high tech as you want. You can weigh and measure and note things down, use apps to log details and calorie counts, or even go as far as to 'tweet what you eat'. There is a *Fixing Dad* App which helps you share your information and progress across your immediate support network.

This initially tedious documenting and recording does something important: it puts the dieter in a position where they are in full control of what they are eating again. It makes them aware of any blips that may have slowed their progress this week and helps them avoid them next week. It helps to explain and make measurable why the bathroom scales are a place of delight one day and an annoyance the next, and it removes some of the frustrating element of chance.

Track your weight

We made Geoff weigh himself at the same time every day, as soon as he got out of bed. We had to keep conditions as similar as possible for each weigh in so he had to be naked and not have had anything to eat or drink. He also had to send us photos of the readout for each measurement. (This also meant having a discreet word with him about not catching his reflection in the glass scales on camera!)

There are many dissenters to this approach. Scales don't measure your body composition, your energy levels, your mental outlook and could lead to disappointments or weight fixations. But in the absence of a better method, this is most people's best option. True, everybody will go through weight fluctuations depending on any number of factors, from bowel contents to hormonal changes, meal patterns, etc. But over time you'll be able to chart trends rather than anomalous ups and downs.

Keep track of your waist circumference too. If that measurement is continuing to get smaller you are certainly losing weight, regardless of any fluctuations on the scales

Measure your setbacks as well as your progress

Being some kind of superhuman who never messes up might well be great, or it might be the most disheartening experience in the world. One of the things that hugely intensifies the buzz of succeeding is when it comes off the back of failure. When our comic book heroes triumph in the end we empathise with them because we have accompanied them through the tense moments when we wondered whether they would make it at all.

Our own efforts are no different. There will be days when all our best intentions collapse. We fall off the wagon so entirely that it seems to have headed way off into the sunset without us. But remember – failure is a vital part of success. It is the means by which you learn to sharpen your techniques in order to get where you want to be.

If your diabetic friend or family member deviates from their new lifestyle overhaul you need to continue to be supportive. If you launch into a full-scale reprimand you will only damage trust, encourage secrecy, compound the sense of failure and isolation. So this is the time to up your support. Make sure you are there to keep them steady.

The long-term, low-carb maintenance plan

Having successfully reversed his type 2 diabetes by losing weight, Geoff has to keep a constant wary eye on his ongoing diet maintenance. Cutting back on carbs, combined with a sensible activity- and age-specific calorie intake, has helped him keep the weight off. But he will always need to remain a low carb-er if he wants to keep his blood glucose under control.

Once you or your diabetic charge are down to a safe and healthy weight after completing the 6 to 8-week plan, you don't need to continue at only 800 calories a day. Just stick to the above guidance for what foods to eat (p.88-9), making sure to steer clear of refined carbs and unnecessary sugars. You might, for example, choose to go on an adapted 5:2, eating 800 calories two days a week and not calorie counting on the other five.

During this phase, you should start to introduce more good fats into your diet as a source of calories. Fat makes you feel fuller for longer so you will find you struggle to eat too much of it, which makes the process somewhat self-correcting. You will become more efficient at burning fat over time, but make sure you keep drinking plenty of water, which is crucial to weight maintenance and your health as a whole.

Get back-up from your doctor

If you are determined to improve your health, you and your diabetic buddy will go the distance. But, just as you wouldn't head off into a blizzard in a bikini, you need to be prepped and sensible. By all means, do your research but, first and foremost, speak to a doctor. There are certainly some people who should not consider embarking on a low-calorie regime (pregnant women and children, for example). There are certain diabetic medications (like gliclazide) which will be affected if you go on a reduced-calorie regime, followed by long-term, low-carb eating, so you need to get the all clear. As mentioned above, your diabetic medication could also become too high for your body's needs as you lose weight, so this will need to be continually monitored.

None of this makes you a medical nuisance. You are part of paving the way towards a new system of preventative, progressive and self-motivated healthcare. Most GPs have the foresight to realise that this approach is a good thing which will save thousands of pounds, and lives, even in the short term – so you should expect encouragement from them. The intermittent monitoring and extra appointment time required early on will certainly pay off in the long run.

Drink water

One last point: be mindful of what you drink. Alcohol was out of the question for Geoff, and should be for you too in those first six to eight weeks, simply to keep your calories low and maximise the nutritional value of what you are taking in. Thereafter it is up to you what you reintroduce, but always be aware of carb and sugar content.

Fruit juices also tend to be high in sugar, so they are not advisable for diabetics. The best drink of all, of course, is – don't groan – water. When you're losing weight you need to make sure you are flushing out toxins effectively, and water really does the trick. Also, in our modern instant-satisfaction consumer society, we aren't very good at distinguishing between thirst and hunger, and sometimes cravings, especially sweet ones, can be satisfied by simply having a glass of water.

Staying hydrated is crucial when you are trying to lose weight, but should also be central to your longer-term health plan.

A cup of hot water is an alternative which weirdly seems to hit much the same spot as a cup of tea or coffee, providing, if not much excitement, a soothing, comforting warmth – plus it hydrates you properly. Try dropping a wedge of ginger in it, a slice of lime, some mint leaves, some berries, a cinnamon stick or whatever you have to hand if you're finding that you need a boost.

Fitness

If the first key element of Anthony and Ian's plan to fix their dad was addressing nutrition, the second was improving his fitness. With Geoff, we found this to be an issue fraught with obstacles.

Finding the right form of exercise

The conventional advice for someone going from doing no exercise to doing some is generally to begin with some light walking. Of course, given the complex problems Geoff experienced with his feet, this wasn't an option. He couldn't drive much weight through his feet, and certainly not the excessive weight that he was carrying then. It seemed as if he was trapped by his own body.

We thought about swimming. However, again, the

circulatory issues in his feet threatened problems – in a germ-ridden swimming pool environment, he would be at risk of infection, and in his case any scratches, cuts or abrasions would struggle to heal.

His personal body image, too, put a question mark over this particular activity. Anxious about the reactions of others, he felt uncomfortable about exposing his body in a public pool. While frustrated at this, his sons had to respect his wishes.

There was only one practical option open to us at this stage and that was cycling. Anthony and Ian resolved that if they kept him on smooth tracks with no inclines, this would limit the weight driving through his feet and any potential strain on his heart.

Some years earlier the family had clubbed together to buy Geoff a bike. It was fairly bespoke as it needed to support his considerable body weight, but for most of those years it ended up supporting only the weight of the gathering dust in Geoff's garage. At last it would come in handy – as is often the case with the contents of Geoff's garage.

Getting started

There were still issues to contend with. Geoff was on medication for his high blood pressure and cholesterol and he also suffered from atrial fibrillation (an irregular heartbeat, particularly common in overweight people). For the most part this was not a huge worry, but it does increase the risk of strokes and heart failure (not to mention dementia, although this wasn't an immediate issue as a consequence of exercise). He was on warfarin to reduce the risk of a stroke but we still had to proceed with extreme caution.

The fitness plan started tentatively. We strapped a heart rate monitor to Geoff's wrist and got him started on gentle warm ups focused mostly on mobilising his joints through slow, careful rotations. When he got on his bike, he and his sons kept a smooth, stately pace over the flatter and quieter roads of Kent. Ian often followed in the car, or drove ahead, so the boys could film how it all went.

Although there is no denying that there were obstacles (such as maintaining the motivation to get up early and head out into whatever the weather had to throw at them)

Geoff: You have me running up and down stairs with my heart going like twenty to the dozen.

Anthony: Yeah, we have to, that's part of saving you. Otherwise you'd be lying on your back eating Wotsits.

Geoff: Yeah… I'd be much more relaxed though.

and sometimes arguments, Geoff's progress was actually faster than we expected. This could have been due to any number of things, but the dual-pronged effect of an improved diet with a steady but progressive exercise plan really seemed to do the trick.

Making progress

The exercise complimented the diet and vice versa: Geoff's new diet was fuelling his body more efficiently, and as he exercised, his body sent much clearer signals about what he should be eating, and about his hydration levels. He had never really experienced this before. In time this took quite a bit of the stress of supervising his every mouthful from his sons. The rules they enforced, which had at first seemed oppressive, were becoming healthy habits that he enjoyed. This was all magnified by the endorphins surging round Geoff's system when he got on his bike and cycled. The spring burst through the bare trees, the summer chased enthusiastically after it and Geoff's skin glowed, his heart pumped, strong and effortlessly.

The signs of improvement could often be seen in the most unexpected ways. Geoff had routine podiatrist checks. Part of these appointments involved removing any dead skin that had accumulated on his feet and checking for circulation. This had never hurt Geoff in any way because he had no feeling in his feet. On one particular day, however, the podiatrist struck gold – or at least the diabetic equivalent. As he carefully removed the layers of dead skin, blood seeped to the surface. This was not some clumsy accident and the podiatrist explained what it meant: Geoff's circulation had improved to such an extent that there was blood flowing through these surface capillaries. It was yet another sign that Geoff was truly coming back from the brink.

Always ambitious, Anthony and Ian decided at this point to ramp up the goals. They knew they needed to keep their dad motivated and they also knew that the goal had to be big enough for him to maintain the serious changes in his lifestyle. They wanted him to start training for the big London-to-Surrey 100-mile ride. Of course, this sort of event is generally the remit of more committed athletes and wouldn't be an appropriate training goal for everyone. But Anthony and Ian were looking for something to really focus Geoff's mind on continuing his exercise. The fact that it was under consideration at all is testament to how effective the last months of diet and exercise had been for him.

When he completed the London-to-Surrey 100 less than a year after that fateful day when Anthony and Ian had sat together and begun devising a plan to fix their dad, Geoff confounded all of our expectations and had astonished the experts. It was a monumental achievement, demonstrating the extent to which Geoff had revolutionised his health.

The true benefits of exercise

Noting all the improvements brought by Geoff's exercise regime, Anthony and Ian went back to see Professor Roy Taylor in Newcastle to give him an update. As they explained how much the exercise had helped in Geoff's battle with the bulge, Professor Taylor smiled patiently. He then gave them some enlightening information on the truth about exercise and weight, information that would prove extremely useful in shaping what they would expect of Geoff's exercise plan as they went forward.

First, Professor Taylor landed a bombshell: that Geoff's weight loss had almost nothing to do with his increased activity and that it was all down to his reduced calorie consumption.

'If you want to lose weight, having become overweight, you can't exercise it away,' Prof Taylor explained.

This seemed worrying: how many times have we

all purged ourselves on exercise equipment following a gastronomic blow out? How often have our trainers hit the tarmac in some form of penance for the hideous hangover we'd woken up with that morning? Was that wasted?

In short: no, it wasn't. Prof Taylor told us that exercise was having huge benefits for Geoff's body – only that weight loss wasn't one of them. From his first training session, the controlled, repetitive movements would have eased synovial fluid through his joints, and his body would begin to feel looser and more agile as his exercise regime progressed. Geoff's heart was getting stronger and more efficient too.

Exercise was also building Geoff's muscle strength to support his skeleton, improving his posture, circulation, mood, bowel function and sleep patterns. It would help protect him against osteoporosis and against further weight gain as his metabolism got going. Additionally, and most crucially for diabetics, building muscle was helping his body become more responsive to insulin.

So there you have it: exercise is not the route to weight loss in itself – to shed the pounds, you have to make changes to your diet, specifically, reduce your consumption. However, there are far-reaching and numerous benefits for both the body and the metabolism of undertaking regular activity. It certainly helps any health plan you decide to undertake. Moreover it is crucial for successfully keeping the weight off once you have lost it.

As we shall see in the next chapter, however, Geoff's achievements in his health revolution were only possible because Anthony and Ian also paid attention to another key area – his mind.

YOUR ROAD MAP

Seek guidance

You must always start any new exercise regime very carefully and under proper guidance. You will need to work out with your GP what exercise is safe for you. It might also be worth running through ideas with a personal trainer or exercise professional. This isn't celebrity stuff for celebrity budgets: your local leisure centre or gym should be able to provide a basic advisory service. For instance, you could book a gym induction and talk through your concerns. It won't tie you to months of compulsory gym membership as most places now have flexible solutions.

Pick your exercise

Don't pick an exercise regime just because you've heard it gets fast results. You need to go for something that you enjoy or that interests you. Consider the following questions for you or your diabetic charge:

- Would I / they prefer indoor or outdoor exercising (such as jogging, cycling etc)?
- Would I / they prefer to train in a solitary or more social environment (e.g. walking alone or going to the gym or to an exercise class)?
- Am I / they a 'stats watcher' or someone that prefers to exercise while developing another skill (e.g. running or weight lifting vs. taking a dance class)?
- Would I / they find certain environments uncomfortable or intimidating (swimming, say, or yoga)?

Likewise, you need to make sure the exercise you choose is safe for you and appropriate to your current fitness levels and health. You will get healthier and stronger with safe training, but if your ideal exercise is mountain climbing, don't be discouraged if you are advised to stick to some gentle hill walking for now.

Your choice of exercise needs to be tailored to your budget. If it involves buying equipment (e.g. a bike) it's a good idea to see what you can borrow to practise on, and so determine whether or not you are going to enjoy it long term.

Finally, always be mindful of any dangers. For diabetics, open wounds – especially on the extremities – are particularly prone to infection due to reduced circulation. An activity such as swimming may prove more problematic in this regard.

When to start

If you are planning to follow the reduced-calorie regime detailed in the previous chapter, you could couple it with the early stages of your exercise programme to get you started. If you or your buddy's current body weight is very high, you may prefer to follow the diet for a couple of weeks before starting to build in an exercise programme.

Either way you need to make an effort to move more – try to build more habitual activity into your everyday life – and start conditioning your body for more regimented exercise. By this, I don't mean that you need to work towards an endurance athlete training schedule; the aim is to move more in a way you enjoy. Take the stairs rather than the lift. Walk to the next bus stop.

Take pleasure in using and mobilising your body as much as you can.

How to start

The key to building fitness is to start slowly. Be sure to lay the groundwork and listen to your body. When you start a new regime you should always be able to hold a conversation while exercising – this is known as 'the talk test'. It is a simple way of ensuring you are not over-exerting your body beyond safe limits. Be aware of feelings of dizziness, nausea or discomfort, and stop if you notice any. Always err on the side of caution and make sure you discuss any issues with your doctor.

Be aware of your posture. A good form will keep your body safe when exercising and ensure all the physical effort is happening in the right places. Also be sure not to neglect stretching, which promotes healing and flexibility in your muscles. Stretching when your muscles are warm after exercising reduces the risk of fainting and decreases the risk of future injury. A local gym instructor will talk you through an appropriate stretching regime for your body and your chosen exercise.

Exercises to get you started

When you are setting out on an exercise regime, don't let the daunting prospect of long cycle rides or endless hikes deter you. You can start small and get used to moving your body in all sorts of ways. These exercises are designed to help your postural awareness and alignment and are a good way to get your muscles going. None of these exercises should cause any physical discomfort or pain. If you are uncomfortable at any point do not continue with the exercise.

Standing crunch

1. Stand just under a foot away from a wall, with your back towards it. Keep your feet flat on the floor, bend your knees and gently lower your back against the wall.
2. Tip your pelvis up slightly so that the length of your spine is pressed against the wall (you should be unable to slip your hand between your back and the wall).
3. Hold for a couple of seconds and then relax the pelvis.
4. Repeat this 8 times, holding the tensed position for varying durations – some short and quick (one to two seconds), some long (eight seconds). You should start to feel warmth in your abdominal muscles.
5. If this exercise feels tough, place your feet closer to the wall.
6. If it feels easy, try it with your arms above your head

(palms forwards, shoulders away from your ears). This requires more force in the abdominal contraction. CAUTION: if you have raised blood pressure you are advised not to exercise with your arms above your head for any prolonged period. If in doubt, stick to the standard exercise only.

Wall press ups

1. Stand within arm's reach of a wall, facing towards it. Place your palms on the wall at shoulder height, shoulder width apart. Your wrists, elbows and shoulders should all be roughly in line.
2. Keeping your core tight and feet still, lower your chest towards the wall. Your elbows should point outwards away from your body as they bend. Remember to feel the full engagement in your core and be aware of the alignment of your spine.
3. Once you are as close to the wall as is comfortable, squeeze your bum/glutes.
4. Push away from the wall until your arms are almost fully extended, a very slight bend still at the elbows.
5. Repeat as many times as is comfortable, stopping one or two reps before you feel fatigued.
6. If you find this exercise difficult, position yourself slightly closer to the wall.
7. For more of a challenge, or to work different muscle

groups, try the same exercise but with your hands wider than shoulder width (therefore requiring more engagement across the chest), or try with the hands closer together (therefore working your triceps more).

Floor knee tucks

1. Lie on your back on the floor and tip your pelvis up slightly so that the length of your spine is pressed against the ground (pay particular attention to the area around your lower back – you should be unable to slip your hand between your back and the floor).
2. With your feet flat on the floor and your knees bent, lift your head and tuck your chin in towards your chest.
3. Alternate lifting each knee in towards your chest, moving slowly and carefully. Keep your abdominal muscles engaged to work this through your core. If you are struggling, ensure your core is engaged; imagine you are bracing for an impact in your stomach – this is the muscle tension you are after.
4. Only repeat as many (or as few) times as is comfortable. It is better to do two or three with good form than 50 with bad form.

Table top knee crunches and leg extensions

1. Position yourself on your hands and knees, with hands directly underneath your shoulders and your back as flat as a table top (doing this in front of a mirror helps). Lift one knee in towards your chest before slowly straightening that leg out behind you.
2. Make sure your hips stay square and in line. You should be able to see the top part of your foot stretching away if you look back between your arms.
3. Repeat until the abdominal muscles, hip flexors and glutes feel nicely warm, as many times as is comfortable, then repeat with the other leg.
4. You can always cushion your knees with a mat, but if it is at all uncomfortable or painful, stop the exercise.

Set goals

You need to set goals but they need to be manageable and progressive. Crucially, these goals should be time-specific: 'By this time next week I will be able to cycle a mile in one ride' / 'By this time next month I will be able to cycle five miles in one go'. And they need to move

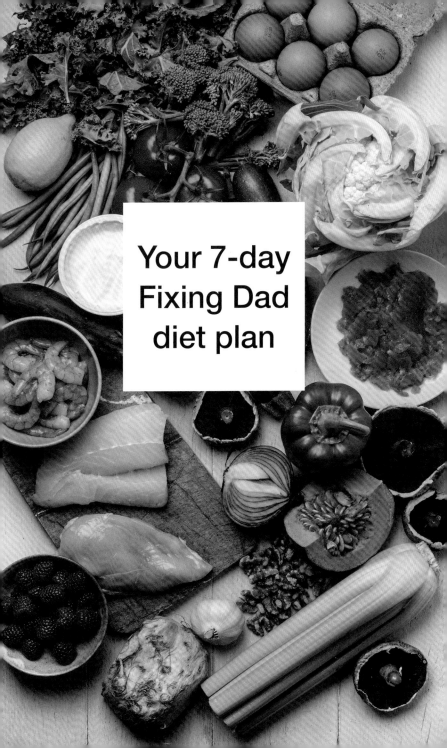

Your 7-day
Fixing Dad
diet plan

Monday

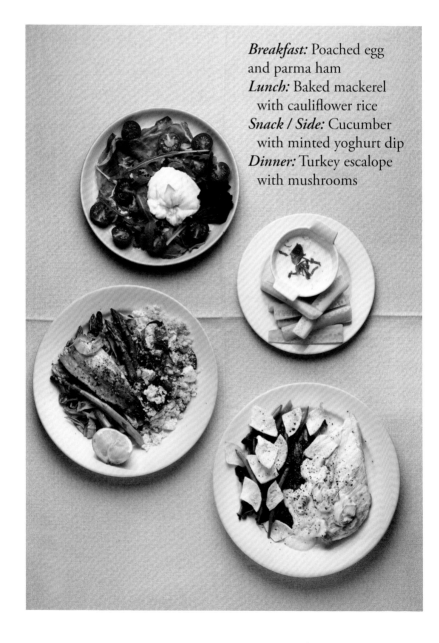

Breakfast: Poached egg
and parma ham
Lunch: Baked mackerel
with cauliflower rice
Snack / Side: Cucumber
with minted yoghurt dip
Dinner: Turkey escalope
with mushrooms

Tuesday

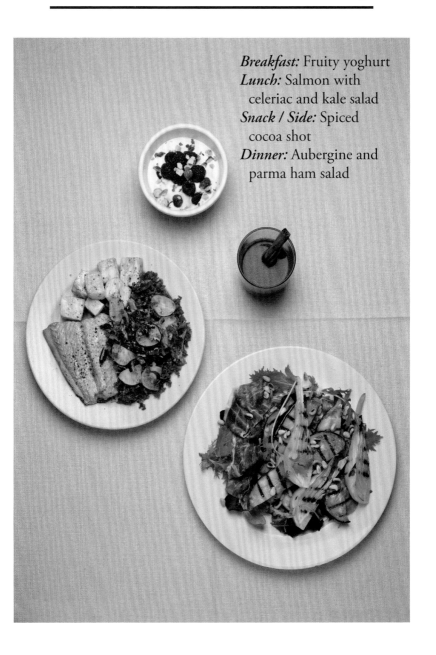

Breakfast: Fruity yoghurt
Lunch: Salmon with
celeriac and kale salad
Snack / Side: Spiced
cocoa shot
Dinner: Aubergine and
parma ham salad

Wednesday

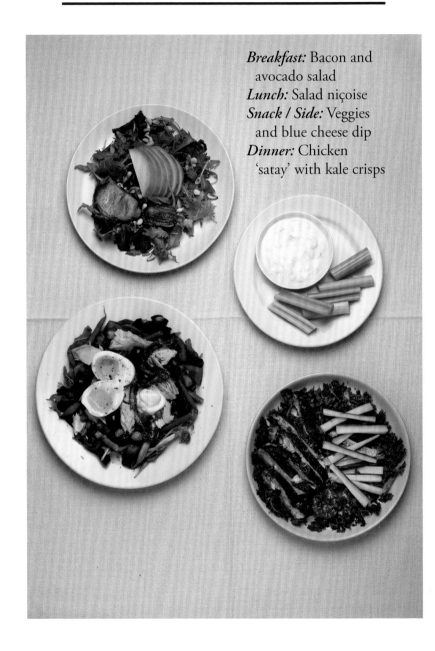

Breakfast: Bacon and avocado salad
Lunch: Salad niçoise
Snack / Side: Veggies and blue cheese dip
Dinner: Chicken 'satay' with kale crisps

Thursday

Breakfast: Scambled egg whites and smoked salmon
Lunch: Chicken with Mediterranean vegetables
Snack / Side: Berry 'smoothie'
Dinner: Broccoli and
 bacon cheese

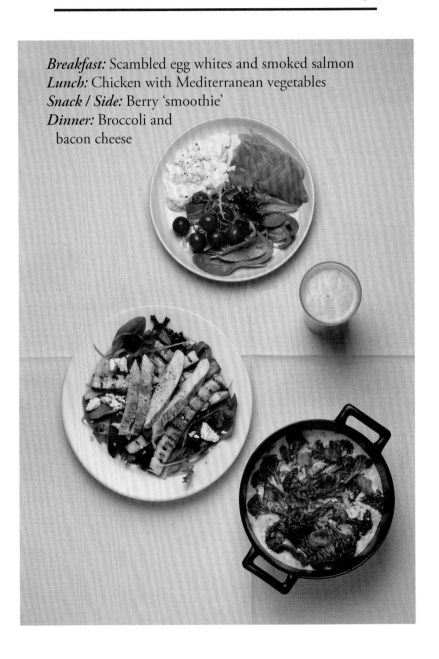

Friday

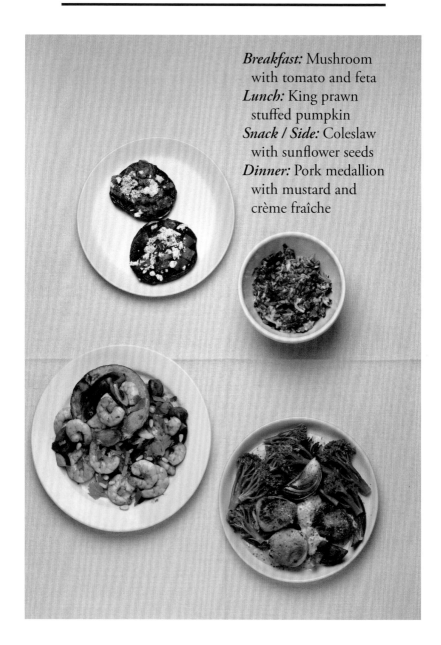

Breakfast: Mushroom with tomato and feta

Lunch: King prawn stuffed pumpkin

Snack / Side: Coleslaw with sunflower seeds

Dinner: Pork medallion with mustard and crème fraîche

Saturday

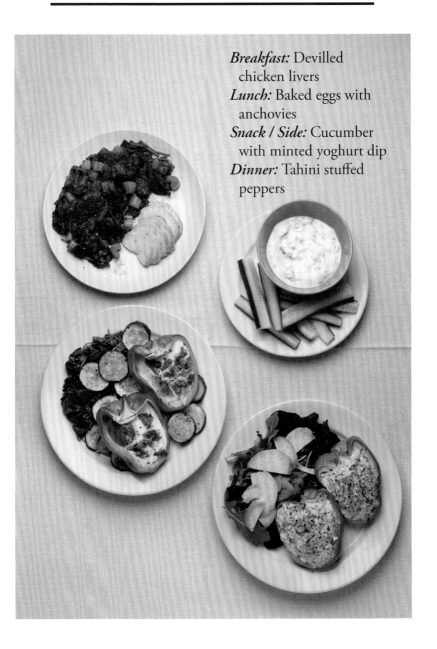

Breakfast: Devilled chicken livers

Lunch: Baked eggs with anchovies

Snack / Side: Cucumber with minted yoghurt dip

Dinner: Tahini stuffed peppers

Sunday

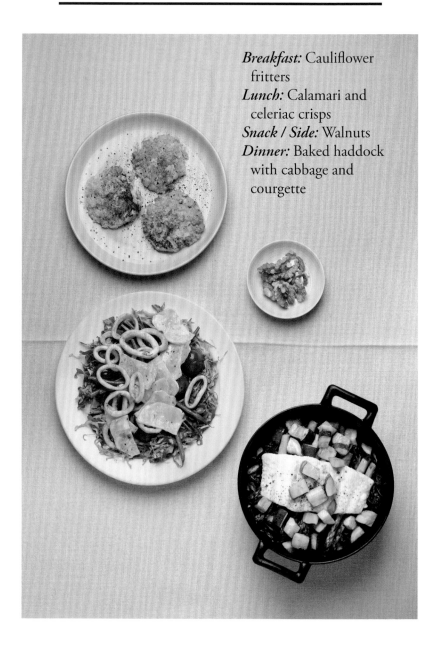

Breakfast: Cauliflower fritters
Lunch: Calamari and celeriac crisps
Snack / Side: Walnuts
Dinner: Baked haddock with cabbage and courgette

forward in safe stages. They need a completion date so you/your buddy can tick them off and feel a tangible achievement.

Goals and targets have to be individual to you, but a possible starting exercise plan might be:

Walking

- Week 1
  A 15-25 minute walk each day with one day off.
- Week 2
  A 15-25 minute walk a day to include one hill with one day off.
- Week 3
  The same walk or one of a similar distance each day to be completed in a faster time, with one day off.
- Week 4 onwards
  Gradually increase the distance, pace, time or resistance (more hills, carrying a light back-pack or using small wrist or ankle weights). By upping the intensity in this way you are more likely to stay safe and working within your progressing fitness levels, without necessarily taking up a huge amount of time.

Cycling

- Week 1-2

    A 30-minute ride every other day. Keep the pace slow and deliberate for the first ten minutes to warm up. For the next 20 minutes you can push a little harder, but only within your comfort zone (remember that you should be able to have a conversation while exercising).
- Week 2-3

    You should begin to feel that you could comfort-ably do a little bit more. After the initial, slower ten minutes, incorporate a hill, or add some extra distance to the route.
- Week 3-4 onwards

    You can up the distance or include an extra hill or two as the weeks go on. But remember the prin-ciple rule: listen to your body. Add what you feel comfortable with and make sure you take your alternate days off.

And again, just to hammer this point home – get your diet and exercise plans approved by a doctor as well as, ideally, a fitness professional. This is not a mere formality. Failure to do so can endanger lives so don't skip it.

Complete goals together

Exercising with your diabetic friend is not essential but it is much more fun. Some of the boys' happiest times during the Fixing Dad project were on the cycle rides they shared together. Doing things as a team builds positive and happy associations until they become habits in their own right. There are very few people who wouldn't benefit from getting out with someone they care about and, if you can get fit and healthy in the process, so much the better.

Other exercise regimes

Both strength training and high intensity interval training are known to have positive effects on insulin resistance and sensitivity but these activities should be explored under the guidance of a professional, ideally one quali-fied to understand insulin readings so as to monitor the changes in your blood glucose levels during exercise.

Strength training needn't be confined to the gym, as you can do a lot without equipment, or use everyday objects around you. For example, you can do push ups or lunges anywhere, and need only a chair or a park bench to perform tricep dips or step ups. Make sure you are prop-erly familiar with good form and safe technique before you launch into anything, and cross-train your muscle groups to avoid problems caused by overtraining any one area. Strength training is great for those days when your body is recovering from your main exercise activity (whether that be cycling, running or whatever routine you choose).

Track progress

Again, it helps to keep a record of how things are coming along. Note down how much you've done and where you've hit your goals. When you look back on your progress diary it will remind you of how far you and/or your supported person have come, especially if this is reinforced with photos and videos. All progress, however small, needs hearty congratulations.

Mind

When Anthony and Ian embarked on their journey to fix their dad's health, they knew there was more to it than just getting his body in better shape. After all, our bodies will only act on the instructions from our brains and, more critically, our minds.

If they thought Geoff's body was scarred from six decades of dangerous habits, there was no telling how many scars he carried in his mind. Thought processes can become habits too, and Geoff's internal monologue had lost most of its positivity over the years.

Geoff's mental scars

We are often told to think positive, to cheer up and believe in ourselves, but being given this advice isn't always helpful – at times, it can be positively counterproductive. Life isn't perfect and despite our best efforts things don't always tick along swimmingly. Geoff had found this to be the case. Bills, worries, health issues – he saw no way off the treadmill. Put simply, Geoff's joy of life had been buried under day-to-day debris. It had led him to believe that his situation was hopeless.

Those mental habits had formed, hardened and calcified; his outlook, his approach to new situations, his belief in what he was worth, what he was capable of... these were all static, unchanging. If his sons had concentrated all their efforts on healing his body alone, they would have missed the root

Ian: You've got this idea in your head that you're not good enough to get anything better.

of the problem. They knew that if they could open up his mind, they would free his body too.

A note on depression

It's important to point out here that, although Geoff was in a bad place mentally, he hadn't reached the stage of full-blown depression. And while the suggested programme offered here may support and be appreciated by someone who is suffering from depression, it is not proposed as a solution to it. An alarmingly high proportion of diabetes patients do suffer from depression, and if you suspect it – diagnosed or not – get help immediately. It is a horrible and potentially fatal condition that should always be taken seriously.

Understanding Geoff

Anthony and Ian decided that to try and get a better understanding of their dad's mentally-ingrained habits, they would take him on a road trip. That way they could observe how he looked at the world and what he focused on when out to enjoy himself. This also allowed them to change his surroundings and get him away from the associations that came with home and work.

One thing they quickly noticed was that Geoff had become lazy and unimaginative about his leisure time and his idea of fun. A day out always revolved around food. A 'treat' was a meal out. Or a snack. Or a side order. Or another meal. Occasionally it was sitting down to watch a film – but that only meant inactivity for a few hours.

The boys wanted to take the general emphasis

off food in particular. The idea was that he could do anything he wanted on a day out. Eating could end up being a *part* of it when necessary but it shouldn't be the main attraction. They wanted to show him that you could build days out around other activities: seeing new places, trying new things, meeting new people.

Getting the focus right

Geoff, Anthony and Ian did all sorts of different bike rides and new activities together, and made some happy memories that they still enjoy recounting. And interestingly Geoff doesn't remember what they had for lunch on those days. The point being this: when you find new sources of enjoyment, other than going for a meal, having a beer at the pub or rewarding yourself with a snack, you will find that you will make those unhealthy habits secondary to other things.

We have already looked at some of the methods that Anthony and Ian used in those early days to get Geoff onside with their fixing plan, in particular their discussions with him about the past, the present and the future, and the interview they conducted in which they uncovered his key impetus for getting healthy – not leaving his family to feel the same sense of guilt and helplessness that he had felt after the death of his mother. These methods were the first steps in helping get his mind on track. Motivation is key. To achieve a personal health revolution the person involved has to truly want it. That motivation has to come from within.

Thereafter it was a matter of getting him to see that a truly positive outcome was achievable.

First, they addressed the issue of blame, the fact that many diabetics burden themselves with guilt for getting this disease. This creates a negative spiral – guilt leads to feelings of worthlessness, which in turn lead to nihilism. By sharing what they had discovered about the rise of the disease in our society – the role of the government, the food industry, the supermarkets and all the clever marketing they employed – Anthony and Ian were able to show Geoff that he needn't view himself as the only culpable party. He was merely part of a much bigger pattern of dysfunction.

Second, the new research into obesity and weight-loss that his sons came across revealed that there *was* a way towards better health – even Geoff could do it. He had achieved so much in his life: he had put others first and had been there for everyone else. Yes, his health was suffering, but he had a lot to be proud of. And his future was in his hands.

When the boys reinforced positive messages with Geoff, they weren't looking only to lead him by the hand – they were trying to get him to internalise those messages, to believe them about himself. He loved his sons, and would never talk to them in the negative way he talked to himself. So why was he treating himself in a way that he wouldn't dream of treating others?

A curveball

Unfortunately, as with any self-improvement plan, there were hiccups. One, in particular, would be major – in terms of Geoff's health, but also his mind.

During an MRI scan undertaken as part of a general medical check to pass him fit for his big 100-mile cycle, Geoff discovered that he had kidney cancer. Yet again we were beyond lucky; the cancer was caught early. Normally kidney cancer is unlikely to be detected until it presents outward symptoms, like blood in the urine. By this point, the chances of beating it will have already fallen.

But, lucky or not, this was tough on Geoff – and for the rest of the family it meant all the positive momentum we had built fell away. Ahead of the surgery to remove the tumour, his sons booked a family holiday in Inverness in the hope of getting him away from it all, and it helped. We all had a great time, although Geoff, probably understandably, fell right off the wagon and his sons realised they would have a difficult job ahead of them to get him back on board.

After the holiday Geoff went up to Guys and St Thomas's Hospital for his surgery. He underwent an operation called a partial nephrectomy to remove the tumour from his right kidney. Thankfully, the operation was a success, but there was a long road of recovery ahead. In his darker moments, Geoff questioned why he had worked so hard to get back in shape only to be felled, however briefly, by this cancer. We meanwhile did our best to reinforce the positives: if Geoff hadn't been at the level of fitness that he had reached and had still been carrying too much weight, he would have been in serious danger when having this operation.

Nonetheless it was a tremendous blow for him and it ate its way into his mind. It was at this point that Anthony and Ian had to retrace their steps to remind themselves of how they had overcome these obstacles before and see if they could employ the same techniques again.

Recovery

Geoff was filled with self-doubt. He'd done so much and what for? He'd ended up being diagnosed with cancer, had to have a big operation, and now his body was sore. He couldn't get out on his bike. He still had to stick to his diet. And there didn't seem to be much joy in anything.

Anthony and Ian now decided to play back that first video interview and remind Geoff of his motivation. They pointed to the records they'd kept of his progress, showed him how his weight had dropped and his circulation improved – all things he had achieved himself. Yes, they'd been there with him, but it was his achievement. They reminded him to congratulate himself, feel proud of how far he had come.

This is one of the reasons that keeping track of progress can be so rewarding: seeing how far you've come and the obstacles you've taken on can really give you a boost when times get tough.

A mindful Geoff

There were other issues to contend with when it came to Geoff's mental state throughout the process, such as stress and anxiety. These had mounted before the fix was underway, back when Geoff feared leaving behind enough money for his family as his health deteriorated. The three of them tried yoga and meditation to escape those negative thought processes. At first

Geoff resisted these activities vehemently, but under the pressure of Anthony and Ian's filming, he gave them a go. It turned out he wasn't as inflexible – physically or mentally – as they had thought, and the yoga went well. Meditation not so much: his breathing was far from zen-like and he found it hard to turn off his galloping brain.

Some things worked, some things didn't. With cycling, though, Geoff developed a new hobby – and hobbies like this can really help reduce stress. In the same way that diet and exercise worked in a virtuous cycle, there was a positive loop between fitness and mind. Exercising relieved stress and released endorphins, and the increase in Geoff's fitness helped him feel more positive about himself too. All of which made him feel more eager to get out and get moving.

YOUR ROAD MAP

When the family embarked on the project of fixing Geoff's health he struggled to make it up a flight of stairs. The things that he ended up doing with his sons – like cycling, hiking, yoga – seemed like impossibilities. None of this just happened, but realising that positive outcomes are achievable is a huge step forwards. Every day that he got soaked out in the rain on his bike in Kent, every time he pushed himself to ride up a hill or another mile, he would have a picture in his head of the positive direction in which he was heading – and was rewarded with the glorious views he could later enjoy.

Talk kindly to yourself

We are all guilty of negative thought patterns. Sometimes these can serve a purpose, but a great deal of the time they just hold us back. If you constantly reinforce all the things you *can't* do, what can never be, what impediments you face, you will stop yourself from trying out the things that you *can* do.

Most of us are lucky enough to have a friend or family member we care about deeply. If we ever heard anyone speaking badly of them or knocking them into the ground, we would certainly pin their ears back. The funny thing is that we are happy to be that objectionable person in our own heads, about ourselves. We scold, belittle and mock ourselves without even realising it.

Make sure you and/or your diabetic friend stand up for yourself, to yourself, in the way that you would for someone you love. You wouldn't think twice about doing it for them and they would do it for you in a blink. Out of respect for them, if not yourself, don't stand for that nonsense any more.

Reshaping your internal voice

Here is an exercise that might help you improve how you talk to yourself.

Keep a notebook with you for a day and divide a few pages in half lengthways. As you go about your daily routine, note down in the left column anything you say to yourself via that internal voice. Don't think too much about the comments – just jot them down as they crop up.

The next day take another look at your list. Notice how your mood changes as you read. Chances are, if you were feeling pretty good before you started, you're probably not any more.

You've probably given yourself all manner of unforgiving reprimands in your time. But now you can take control. Count the number of times you use core negative words such as: 'can't', 'won't', 'don't', 'not', 'no'. Pretty often, right? And when you're feeling low, you need positivity, not negativity. So, in the second column, write down how you could rephrase each sentence to be more constructive.

This isn't as difficult as you might think. To give some guidance, here are a few examples we collected when we heard Geoff blurt out something that came from his negative internal voice:

Negative statement: *'A hundred miles! I don't think so somehow!'*

Positive alternative: *'A hundred miles sounds like a long way. I can start training and see how far I get. I would be so proud to even get close.'*

Remember that the end goal for an activity such as Geoff's 100-mile ride isn't what's important – it's the work that's put in that counts. The last sentence in the positive alternative above is where the real power lies: you are creating a picture in your head and a sensation in your body of the feeling of achievement, whatever the final outcome.

Negative statement: *'No one is going to listen to me. What do I know?'*
Positive alternative: *'I may not have any medical qualifications, but I know a lot about being a patient and some of that may be helpful to others in my position.'*

The second statement here was Geoff's response to the idea of speaking at conferences about his diabetes. It was certainly a challenge getting someone who wasn't happy with public speaking to open up to the idea. The key was to shift the focus away from Geoff's doubts about what he couldn't offer, onto what he could, and onto those who might benefit from it.

Negative statement: *'I'm not eating that… thing.'*
Positive alternative: *'That's not something I would*

normally want to try but I could see what it tastes like. If it tastes the way I suspect then I'll just spit it out – but if it's good it may become a new favourite.'

Trying to reframe your thoughts isn't easy. Remind yourself of how small the cost will be if something new doesn't work out (such as Geoff needing to spit out the food if it does taste bad), and compare that with what you stand to gain if it does (in this case finding a new favourite food, or a food that opens up a new avenue to healthy eating). Thinking in terms of making even the littlest things sound possible has a knock-on effect on the bigger things later.

Reducing stress

Stress is a significant factor when it comes to insulin levels and weight gain. It can be brought on because of your environment, your private and professional life or your sleep patterns, to name but a few causes.

You might have a few methods of your own for de-stressing that you have tried before, such as zoning out in front of the telly, taking a wander around the shops, or listening to music. You know the ones that help and the ones that don't. Geoff found that working with his hands took his mind off things that were troubling him. Try looking for things that keep your brain and your body busy. If you also have something to show for it at the end (as Geoff did with cycling, or with DIY) it will continue to reinforce your new direction. Find a project and have some fun with it.

As we've seen, Geoff wasn't one for meditation, and the idea may not suit you either. Here's an exercise that did work for Geoff, however; a sort of physical meditation aimed simply at creating a pleasant relaxed feeling in your body. The exercise takes about three to five minutes but you could extend it.

All movements must be gentle and slow with gradual and comfortable increases to your range of motion. You should not feel any pain or discomfort at any time – if you do, stop. It helps to do this in front of a full-length mirror so that you can keep an eye on your physical alignment.

Rotations and stretches to help reduce stress

1. Stand with your feet hip-width apart and your head and spine aligned. Slowly lower your chin to your chest so you can feel a gentle stretch in the back of your neck. Then roll your head around to the left so that your ear drops towards your left shoulder, stretching the opposite side of your neck. Roll your head back to the middle, chin to chest. Repeat on the other side. Do this routine a couple of times until you feel a softening of the neck muscles.

2. Gently move your head up and down like an exag-

gerated nod, chin down to chest and then up.
Don't drop the back of your head too much and
work only within the natural movement of the joint.

3. Lift your shoulders up towards your ears (like a big
    shrug) and lower them down. Repeat several times
    to release tension.

4. Rotate your shoulders in slow, circular movements.
    Start by bringing your shoulders forward and then
    scooping them up towards your ears. Roll them
    back (as though squeezing your shoulder blades
    together) and lower them round to complete the
    loop. Do this 6-8 times before repeating in the
    opposite direction.

5. Clasp your hands together, interlocking your fingers.
    Roll your hands in a circular motion 6-8 times one
    way before repeating in the opposite direction.

6. Place your feet hip-width apart and put your hands
    on your hips. Gently move your hips in a circle.
    Start by shifting your hips to the left before pushing
    your bottom backwards. Move your hips round to
    the right and then bring your pelvis forward, so as
    to complete the full circle. Do this 6-8 times before
    repeating in the opposite direction.

7. Gently bend your knees and, keeping your back
    straight, rest your hands on your thighs – above the
    knees not on the knees. Slowly and carefully lower
    yourself by bending your knees (not your back),

before returning to your starting position. Repeat 6-8 times or as many times as is comfortable.

8. If your joints are good you can stay in this position and make small, circular movements with your knees (rotating both together, side by side), 6-8 times clockwise before repeating anticlockwise.

9. Holding onto a surface or wall for balance if necessary, stand on one foot and rest the ball of other on the ground. Gently circle the ankle joint by rotating the heel one way (6-8 times or as many as comfortable) and then repeat in the other direction. Repeat with the other foot.

Whether you do this in the morning, evening or both it is worth making time for. It helps your balance, freedom of movement and flexibility and it gives your mind a welcome break from the usual brain buzzing.

Find new rewards (and try new things)

When you listen out for it, you hear it everywhere: 'I might treat myself to a bit of cake, why not?' Yes, 'why not?' – but also 'why?' It can easily become a habit to reward yourself with food – even when you're not actually hungry – because it's gratifying and doesn't take much thought. Your mind might see it as a treat but if you're a type 2 diabetic it is anything but a treat for your body. Look out for other forms of gratification: phoning someone that you haven't spoken to for ages, planning a day out with some friends, picking up an old hobby or trying something completely new. Make it something that supports your plans, something you can do easily. Suddenly you've started a new habit.

Change your surroundings

Sometimes it takes a new environment to make real changes. The Whitingtons went on a tight-budget road trip to get Geoff out of his home environment and open his mind to new things. You needn't go to the same lengths, although putting in some time to change the scenery can really help.

In the old days, wherever he was going, for Geoff the primary concern was where he would eat. His sons got him to turn this idea of a 'day out' on its head.

When you go somewhere new, take a healthy lunch with you and focus on exploring, or just doing something active – it can become a reward of its own.

If you go further afield in your search for a new scene, just be sure to plan your trip thoughtfully. Try and stick to breaks that support what you are doing and already achieving. Test out your healthy habits in the new environment and challenge yourself to see how robust they are. Self-catering holidays beat all-you-can-eat buffet hotels in this regard, as do holidays centered around activity and sightseeing rather than flopping on a beach.

Expect setbacks

Obstacles – big, small and seemingly insurmountable – will always crop up. As obstacles go, Geoff's cancer was a big one, and we were lucky to have caught it when we did – not everyone is. Some cancers have been linked to lifestyle and factors such as excess weight (kidney cancer now being one of the cancers linked to obesity), but there was no way of knowing whether it played a part in Geoff's condition.

After going through everything he did, we couldn't blame him for lapsing back into some of his old, unhealthy ways; the aim became not to allow him to undo all the good he had done.

Whether your setbacks come in the form of argu-ments and rifts, collapses in motivation or resolve, or full scale medical emergencies, by now you will be coming to realise what the valuable lesson is here: ultimately, the obstacle isn't important, it's more about how we find our way past it. Your attitude and approach to setbacks will massively shape how you deal with them.

Getting back on track

It is easier said than done to beat a setback or get back on track when you've let things slip. Don't be hard on yourself. Look back over the motivations that got you going on this health journey. Feel proud of yourself, and get inspired again.

PART 4:

THE AFTER MAN

Going forward

Hopefully by now you are starting to form an idea of how you could adapt Anthony and Ian's plan for your own particular set of circumstances. Hopefully you are also starting to see that most of the challenges ahead are more perceived than real and that there is a way around them.

You may even be in full swing and seeing results already.

But then what? What happens once you've got yourself or the person you are supporting back to good health and the job is now maintaining that? You can't keep losing weight or cycling up steeper and steeper hills.

> **Anthony:** Of course, there are barriers to fixing our health, but the barriers should never be ourselves.

It is at this point – the fear of the plateau – where Anthony and Ian eventually found themselves with

Geoff. They could safely say he had recovered from the depths of ill health, and with it their filming project was over (now requiring an edit to turn it into an hour-long film). Yes, everyone was still there for Geoff, but to an increasing extent he was on his own, to continue as he saw fit.

Geoff's health revolution had been so effective that, under medical supervision, he had been able to come off all of his diabetes medication. He still had to test his blood sugars routinely and visit the diabetic clinic to keep an eye on his foot health but, certainly from a pharmaceutical point of view, Geoff was diabetes free. He even received a consultant's letter which, under the heading 'Type 2 Diabetes', simply said: 'Resolved'. However, as with the continued need for monitoring, we knew that there was still the potential for the mechanisms that went wrong before to go wrong again if they weren't kept in check.

To some extent, of course, Geoff had been on this journey long enough for most of the habits to have stuck. He was much clearer on what he was and wasn't allowed to eat and he really enjoyed his new exercise regimes, the cycling in particular. But just as progress in the right direction can creep slowly along without you noticing a difference, the same is true of slipping backwards.

This is a risk that has to be faced, whether you

are the subject of a successful health revolution, or a supporter. Geoff needed to know how to go out for a pub lunch and not go crazy on his previous scale. He needed to know how to order from a menu and select things that weren't going to play havoc with his blood glucose levels (which primarily meant staying off those big carbs).

Anthony and Ian still checked in with Geoff regularly, and Geoff was keen to avoid regressing. But little changes, for whatever reasons, did start to occur. Perhaps his sons' rules became more lenient when left to Geoff's management. Perhaps he felt such a long way from that old life that dipping the occasional non-ulcerated toe back into an old behaviour seemed harmless. When there was a lapse, Geoff resolved, as usual, to get back on top of it tomorrow – but resolve and intention amount to nothing without committed action.

There were a couple of things that the boys encouraged Geoff to put in place to help himself stay on track: to get on the scales *every morning*, as he had been before, thus reaffirming the habit that got him to focus on what he ate, and what he was going to eat over the course of the day. And to continue his food diary.

But Geoff came to see the scales once more as a site of disappointment when he was aware he had let his good habits slip. So he preferred to bury his head in the sand and wait to weigh himself when he felt they would present better news.

Without anyone noticing, Geoff put on nearly a stone over the Christmas period. With his blood sugars back up, he had to go back to one metformin a day. This should have been sobering for him, but in his view one was better than the four he had been on previously, so the odd indulgence was now permissible. This was exactly what his sons had feared – Geoff had found excuses to take his eye off the ball. In his view he was exercising more these days so it was OK for him to eat a bit more. In reality he wasn't exercising as much, and many of his food choices, while massively better than his old ones, were not ideal. Anthony and Ian were frustrated by this regression.

Letting things slip

Unfortunately, the sort of relapse in behaviour Geoff went through is horribly common among recovered type 2 diabetics. Over the course of working with Geoff, and at various campaign events devised to raise awareness of this route out of type 2 diabetes, we met many fellow sufferers who had found themselves in a similar situations. When driven by the impetus of worsening ill-health, or amputations, or death, sufferers had no shortage of motivation to do everything they could to get better. Once they got there, however, it was all too easy to get complacent and let the good times roll.

There are ways, as Geoff and the family found, to straighten things out, and it is true to say that those recovered diabetics we met who were coping best with their 'new normal' were the ones who had settled right into their new way of life and almost forged a new identity for themselves in the process – a lifestyle built around good habits and healthy eating.

In the end, it didn't take a lot for Geoff to get back on top of it all again. In fact, it required just a couple of gentle prompting conversations with his sons. As with the methods mentioned in the chapter on mind, Anthony and Ian could remind Geoff of all he had achieved, and of his motivations at the outset. They reminded him to think a day at a time again, to look for alternatives to turning immediately to food when feeling peckish, such as having a black coffee or a glass of water, or occupying his mind with other things. He introduced a couple of low-calorie days each week which helped to reset his thinking about appetite. He set himself some new goals and revisited old ones (one of which was training for another big, 100-mile cycle ride). He got back to framing things more positively in his mind again too.

And this time it stuck. These days he has truly accepted that his low-carb diet and more active lifestyle are not simply part of a one-off project. They are who he is now and they are here to stay. He rarely gives that a thought because it has become his new normal and *that* is a major triumph.

YOUR ROAD MAP

As crucial a point in this whole process as getting started is returning to a new 'normal'. This is the point when you've done your low-carb or low-calorie/low-carb diet, the weight has fallen off, you are off most, if not all, of your diabetic medication (having been reducing it under medical supervision) and you can get on with rebuilding your life after diabetes. Sliding back down the mountain that you have just put so much effort into climbing is the worst thing you can do as you'll only have to climb up it again – or succumb once more to illness.

Stick together

This is a time when, as a supporter, you need to be

there as much as ever, if not more. Seeing the person you have helped glowing with vitality and positivity is the most rewarding part of this whole process, but it is not the end. It is crucial that the support doesn't stop here, even though their dieting may not need to be as extreme as in those first six to eight weeks, and the goals may not feel quite as progressive.

If you are the person revolutionising your own health you may feel like you've made it – and you really have – but it isn't over yet. Don't be afraid to seek the continued support of friends and family. Keep them with you until you are confident that you can face it down alone. Believe me, it will do you all good: your newfound health and (possibly shared) positive activities reaffirming a whole new lifestyle for everyone.

Maintain your goals

With the daily horrors of ill health far behind you, it is much harder to stay motivated. At this point you need to find new and renewed incentives to stay healthy, other than just feeling better.

Think about why you set out on this course, and what you were, and still are, trying to avoid happening to your health. Review your progress, take pride in it, let it boost your positive viewpoint. Like Geoff, you could find new exercise goals – either new targets or new forms of exercise altogether. Most importantly, keep an eye on those eating habits: make low-carb and healthy eating (including using the recipe ideas featured in the final section of this book) part of who you are. And if you need an extra kick, incorporate a low-calorie day or two into your week.

Keep measuring

Imperfect as they are, you need the scales. You may be able to stop weighing and measuring everything you are eating (by now you'll have a good idea of what sensible portion sizes look like) but you still need to weigh yourself most days.

The scales are not going to give you an accurate measure of your overall health and happiness but they are going to help you stay on track. A couple of pounds here and there is nothing to beat yourself up over – but it is important not to ignore longer-term weight gain trends. If you're the kind of person who puts off weighing yourself until the reading is likely to be one you're happy with then you could well end up avoiding the scales forever. Weigh yourself daily to sharpen your focus. Allow yourself to get a buzz from keeping your weight level. The straight line on a healthy weight graph is the sure and certain path of being well.

Enjoy your hard work

In the early days, dragging his bike out of the garage when he felt tired, Geoff found cycling a chore, something he needed to get done to keep his sons off his back. Now he is in better shape and more confident, it is how he chooses to unwind, how he finds focus and even how he celebrates time off.

The way you frame something in your mind is very important. Back when Geoff's body was ailing, everything was an effort – but that changed. Enjoy the things you are able to do now that you couldn't do before. Set aside some time each day when you think about the improvements in your life and health, however minor. If you attach this thought process to another activity you do every day (cleaning your teeth, feeding the cat, etc) you won't forget. If you reinforce those positive changes every day by being mindful of them or being grateful for them, you will be less likely to slip back into unhealthy practices. You've worked hard, you should enjoy it.

And what about the supporters? Sometimes it may feel like a thankless task, and you may wonder why on earth you are bothering. One of the most powerful things you can do to reinforce your efforts is to remember that you've engaged in this whole process out of love. Without this, you would have given up long ago. As you go about your daily routine, consider all the great memories and precious moments you have nurtured that you might otherwise never have had. This is the beautiful view at the top of the mountain you have just climbed.

The future

The last piece of advice from Geoff's journey: keep the goals going. Keep them small, medium and large; short-, medium- and long-term. Cover all the bases of mind, fitness and nutrition and get yourself, in every respect, back in the best shape of your life. Who knows? Tough as your journey has been or will be, you may inspire those around you.

And it may go even further than that, as it did for Geoff. He has talked at international diabetes conferences to try and increase awareness about the realities for patients with type 2. He has spoken to audiences of the need to be spurred into action, and the sorry fact that, for too many people, such a point comes too late. He has seen how the professionals and medics treating this disease have sometimes been swept up in the wave of pessimism, or apathy, that surrounds it. When Geoff, too, had doubts along the way, he could remind himself that his efforts might just inspire others, even just one person, to make changes in their life that could save them some suffering.

Geoff knew, as he stood at that lectern at the EASD Conference in Croatia, that he was not a natural public speaker, but Anthony and Ian were close at hand and were willing him on.

When he had agreed to do these talks, Geoff had decided he would be the dad his sons looked up to, the one who wouldn't be beaten without a fight. And, as he looked down at his speech, with its underlines, block capitals, prompts and pauses, he knew that one man in a sea of statistics counted for something. If he, Geoff, could banish this disease from his own body, then he could play a part in showing others how to do the same.

He knew all the words he wanted to say and they came out as he intended – but they sounded different in that room compared to when he had been practising them in the hotel. They sounded different because this time they came from somewhere else. This time they came from his heart. The audience beamed back at him and applauded enthusiastically. Some said later that Geoff's speech was the highlight of the conference; others that it was stories like his that got them out of bed in the morning.

Geoff could only smile sheepishly while his sons swelled with pride. It was their dad on that stage, their dad being applauded, who had spoken out and wanted to make a difference, when not so long ago he had only been able to wring his hands or shrug his shoulders. The three of them knew that it was down to the difference between standing alone and standing together.

When Geoff had doubted himself, his sons believed in him. We all did, and whatever it was that got Geoff to where he was – belief, hope, science or good old-fashioned luck – we as a family are grateful every day to have this man still with us and for the memories that our collective mission to reclaim his health has given us. As an all-round family adventure I would heartily recommend it.

YOUR ROAD MAP

Don't be scared of change

Remember the saying, 'If you always do what you always did, you will always get what you always got.' This could not be more true here.

This journey is going to change your life. You will be healthier, happier, better supported and more purposeful. BUT – this will require a shake up in your life, and/or the life of the person you are looking to support. This shake up will affect everything, from your habits to your daily menus, your wardrobe (you will need better fitting clothes as your old ones get baggy), and, most importantly, your view of yourself. People will challenge you and try to pull you back to the person they knew you to be, but resist and persist.

Slowly but surely those around you will accept who you (or your diabetic charge) are becoming. If you are the much-needed supporter in this process, join in. It makes it fun to go through these things together and it forges bonds between you in a way that few other things can.

Take control

This whole process has a lot to do with control. If it is your own health you are revolutionising, you will need a good grip on your diet and exercise. You will also need to take control of your thought processes, the things you say to yourself in your head. Your mind will dictate how your body responds.

When it comes to moments of frailty, when, say, you may fancy a tub of ice cream or a pint of beer, ask yourself a straightforward question: do you want that treat as much as you want your health back? Reframe your mind and stay focused on your end goal, however far away it may seem.

If you are the supporter, be aware that there will be times when you may need to step in and take charge, to help hold back the tide of people offering treats and calories. You may have to reinforce your buddy's willpower. You may need to remind them of their goals and their progress so far. Give them the confidence to push themselves a bit beyond their comfort zone. Chances are that if you are the one helping them, you probably know them very well, so be confident in your ability to gauge what prompts they will respond to best.

Bon voyage

We all like a happy ending but whether or not we get one does depend so much on ourselves. As far as this book goes, my sign-off may or may not be a welcome one, depending on how you choose to take it.

Here's the truth: better habits can be enforced and big changes can be achieved over as little as two months. But if you truly want to take control of your long-term health these changes need to stick – for life. And by 'life' I don't just mean 'forever'; I mean those choices that you make every day to support and sustain *your life*.

Get started, keep going and get well and I would love to know how you're getting on.

Jen xx

PART 5:

RECIPES AND MEAL PLANS

Geoff's diet plan

What follows in this section are the four weekly meal plans that we devised for Geoff for those first reduced-calorie weeks – they are filled with only good ingredients, all are low-carb, and total around 800 calories a day. You can simply repeat the four weeks to make up your six or eight low-cal weeks, or mix around the recipes to include more of your favourites.

The recipes are so simple that even a reluctant, kitchen-phobic Geoff Whitington could cook them – and do the minimal washing up involved. In order to help you beat your diabetes, or help someone close to you do what Geoff did, everything is spelled out, no fuss. And after the early, low-calorie weeks have passed, these same recipes can be adapted for sticking to a gentler, longer-term, low-carb diet. No longer needing to watch your calories, you can include enough healthy fats for satiety.

Other useful information sources

If you're looking for more ideas along the way, use an app that tracks calorie intake (*My Fitness Pal* is very good) and look up recipes that follow a Mediterranean-style diet low in carbohydrates. If you want to make any substitutions just make sure you stay within your calorie limits in those first six to eight weeks. You can find more recipes on the *Fixing Dad App*, which offers full nutritional support. Also, Dr Michael Mosley has written an excellent book on this subject called *The 8-Week Blood Sugar Diet*, which includes lots of recipes and suggestions. He too has worked closely with Prof Roy Taylor (and mentions Geoff's story in his book).

Log your weight on an app as you go along too. The ones with graphs are great because you get a much more satisfying picture of your weight loss when you see the line going down.

We have included weekly shopping lists with the meal plans but you can devise your own based on the things you like best. There is a lot of veg in every recipe but you need to make sure you get your daily protein requirement (40-50g).

While the shopping lists may look quite lengthy,

many of the same ingredients are reused over the weeks. The chances are that you may have a lot of them at home already, and you'll find this increasingly the case as the weeks go on. The lists can therefore also help you reorganise what you have in the cupboard or freezer. Spare bits of meat and fish can be frozen for another week and this will save buying more in future. Remember that the quantities in an individual recipe are small.

It's easy, too, to keep things flexible. With a little weighing, measuring and a bit of maths you can substitute different ingredients – just make sure you avoid refined carbs and, if you are substituting vegetables, stick to surface-growing ones. Use root veg like carrot and parsnips sparingly as they are quite high in carbohydrate. Celeriac is OK in smaller quantities, as it is slightly lower-carb and full of flavour. Remember that spices and herbs are your friends when it comes to mixing up the flavours.

A guide to what will need to be washed up is included with each recipe, listing anything used in the cooking (pans, mixing bowls etc). Chopping boards, plates and knives and forks are not listed to avoid repetition, as these will invariably be required in each case.

Most recipes serve one as that's what we had to work out for Geoff. Simply increase the ingredients if you are cooking for two or cooking in bulk (or, of course, if you have completed the low-calorie phase). A few recipes serve two, simply because they are easier to cook in bulk. If you are cooking for one, you can always refrigerate or freeze portions for another day.

Geoff likes to be prepared for all eventualities and likes it when things are planned meticulously. Of course, this doesn't fit with everybody (his sons for example!). So we have made sure there is room to mix things up a bit if you choose to. This is why **all breakfasts are 130 calories each, all lunches and suppers are 260 calories, and all snacks/sides are 60 calories**. You can then swap meals around as you choose, and still have 90 calories spare for milk in tea or coffee (about 200ml of semi-skimmed over the day, or 70ml of whole milk), or an extra side with your main.

Give it a go – and good luck!

Week 1 – Menu Plan

	Breakfast 130 cal	Lunch 260 cal
Mon	Poached egg and Parma ham p.187	Baked mackerel with cauliflower rice p.192
Tue	Fruity yoghurt p.179	Salmon with celeriac and kale salad p.194
Wed	Bacon and avocado salad p.181	Salad niçoise p.196
Thu	Scrambled egg whites and smoked salmon p.182	Chicken with Mediterranean vegetables p.198
Fri	Mushroom with tomato and feta p.184	King prawn stuffed pumpkin p.200
Sat	Devilled chicken livers p.185	Baked eggs with anchovies p.189
Sun	Cauliflower fritters p.186	Calamari and crisps p.199

Snacks / Sides 60 cal	Dinner 260 cal
Cucumber with minted yoghurt dip p.222	Turkey escalope with mushrooms p.208
Spiced cocoa shot p.221	Aubergine and parma ham salad p.209
Veggies and blue cheese dip p.219	Chicken 'satay' with kale crisps p.212
Berry 'smoothie' p.220	Broccoli and bacon cheese p.214
Coleslaw with sunflower seeds p.218	Pork medallion with mustard and crème fraîche p.211
Cucumber with minted yoghurt dip p.222	Tahini stuffed peppers p.207
Walnuts 10g p.222	Baked haddock with cabbage and courgette p.206

Week 1 – Shopping List

Fruit and Vegetables

Asparagus
Aubergines
Avocados
Basil
Broccoli
Cauliflower
Celeriac
Celery
Cherry tomatoes
Coriander, fresh
Courgettes
Cucumber
Fennel
Garlic, bulb
Green beans
Kale
Lemons

Mint
Mixed salad leaves
Mushrooms
Peppers, green and red
Portabello mushrooms
Pumpkin (or crown/prince
  squash)
Radishes
Raspberries (or blueberries)
Red cabbage
Red onions
Spinach
Spring greens
Spring onions
Tomatoes
White cabbage

Dairy

Blue cheese
Butter
Cheddar cheese
Crème fraiche
Eggs, large (about 8)

Feta
Parmesan
Ricotta
Yoghurt, natural full fat

164

Meat and fish

Back bacon
Calamari, fresh
Chicken breast fillets,
  skinless
Chicken livers
Haddock
King prawns

Mackerel fillets
Parma ham (or Serrano)
Pork medallions
Salmon fillets
Smoked salmon
Turkey escalope (lean,
  thin steaks)

Cupboard

Anchovy fillets
Black olives
Black pepper
Capers
Cayenne pepper
Chili powder
Chinese five spice
Cinnamon sticks
Cocoa powder, unsweetened
Dijon Mustard
Hazelnuts
Mayonnaise
Mustard
Oil (olive or coconut)

Paprika
Peanut butter
  (100% peanut)
Pecans
Pine nuts
Psyllium husk powder
Salt
Soy sauce
Sunflower seeds
Tahini
Tuna (tinned in springwater)
Tumeric
Walnuts

	Breakfast 130 cal	Lunch 260 cal
Mon	Scrambled egg and avocado p.183	Kedgeree p.204
Tue	Blueberry 'pancake' p.188	Steak and (sort of) chips p.190
Wed	Coconut porridge p.180	Aubergine and spinach bake with mozzarella p.202
Thu	Poached egg and Parma ham p.187	Baked mackerel with cauliflower rice p.192
Fri	Fruity yoghurt p.179	Salmon with celeriac and kale salad p.194
Sat	Bacon and avocado salad p.181	Salad niçoise p.196
Sun	Scrambled egg whites and smoked salmon p.182	Chicken with Mediterranean vegetables p.198

Snacks / Sides 60 cal	Dinner 260 cal
Spiced cocoa shot p.221	Crab cakes and green salad p.216
Coleslaw with sunflower seeds p.218	Poached eggs and mushrooms p.213
Berry 'smoothie' p.220	Courgette pizzas with salmon fillet p.210
Cucumber with minted yoghurt dip p.222	Turkey escalope with mushrooms p.208
Spiced cocoa shot p.221	Aubergine and parma ham salad p.209
Veggies and blue cheese dip p.219	Chicken 'satay' with kale crisps p.212
Berry 'smoothie' p.220	Broccoli and bacon cheese p.214

Week 2 – Shopping List

Fruit and Vegetables

Asparagus
Aubergines
Avocados
Basil
Blueberries
Broccoli
Cauliflower
Celeriac
Celery
Cherry tomatoes
Coriander, fresh
Courgettes
Cucumber
Fennel
Garlic, bulb
Green beans

Kale
Lemons
Mint
Mixed salad leaves
Mushrooms
Peppers, green
Portabello mushrooms
Radishes
Raspberries (or blueberries)
Red cabbage
Spinach
Spring greens
Thyme
Tomatoes
White cabbage

Dairy

Blue cheese
Butter
Cheddar
Crème fraîche
Feta
Eggs, large (about 12)

Mozzarella
Parmesan
Ricotta
Yoghurt, natural full fat

Meat and fish

Back bacon

Beef escalope (thin,
  lean steaks)

Skinless chicken breast fillets

Crab meat, fresh or tinned

Mackerel fillet

Parma ham (or Serrano)

Salmon fillets

Smoked salmon

Turkey escalope

Cupboard

Anchovy fillets

Black olives

Black pepper

Capers

Chinese five spice

Cinnamon (sticks or
  powder)

Cocoa powder, unsweetened

Coconut flour

Coconut milk, tinned,
  full fat

Curry powder

Dijon mustard

Hazelnuts

Mayonnaise

Mustard

Oil (olive or coconut)

Peanut butter
  (100% peanut)

Pecans

Pine nuts

Psyllium husk powder

Salt

Soy sauce

Sunflower seeds

Tomatoes, tinned

Tuna, tinned in springwater

Vanilla extract

	Breakfast 130 cal	Lunch 260 cal
Mon	Mushroom with tomato and feta p.184	King prawn stuffed pumpkin p.200
Tue	Devilled chicken livers p.185	Baked eggs with anchovies p.189
Wed	Cauliflower fritters p.186	Calamari and crisps p.199
Thu	Scrambled egg and avocado p.183	Kedgeree p.204
Fri	Blueberry 'pancake' p.188	Steak and (sort of) chips p.190
Sat	Coconut porridge p.180	Aubergine and spinach bake with mozzarella p.202
Sun	Poached egg and Parma ham p.187	Baked mackerel with cauliflower rice p.192

Snacks / Sides 60 cal	Dinner 260 cal
Coleslaw with sunflower seeds p.218	Pork medallion with mustard and crème fraîche p.211
Cucumber with minted yoghurt dip p.222	Tahini stuffed peppers p.207
Walnuts 10g p.222	Baked haddock with cabbage and courgette p.206
Spiced cocoa shot p.221	Crab cakes and green salad p.216
Coleslaw with sunflower seeds p.218	Poached eggs and mushrooms p.213
Berry 'smoothie' p.220	Courgette pizzas with salmon fillet p.210
Cucumber with minted yoghurt dip p.222	Turkey escalope with mushrooms p.208

Week 3 – Shopping List

Fruit and Vegetables

Asparagus
Aubergines
Avocados
Basil
Blueberries
Broccoli
Cauliflower
Celeriac
Celery
Cherry tomatoes
Coriander, fresh
Courgettes
Garlic, bulb
Green beans
Lemons
Mint
Mixed salad
Mushrooms
Peppers, green
Portabello mushrooms
Pumpkin (or crown/prince squash)
Raspberries (or blueberries)
Red cabbage
Red onions
Spinach
Spring greens
Spring onions
Tomatoes
Thyme
White cabbage

Dairy

Butter
Cheddar
Crème fraîche
Eggs, large (about 14)
Feta
Mozzarella
Parmesan
Ricotta
Yoghurt, natural full fat

172

Meat and fish

Beef escalope

Chicken livers

Crab meat, fresh or tinned

Calamari, fresh

Haddock fillet

King prawns

Mackerel fillet

Parma ham (or Serrano)

Pork medallions

Salmon fillet

Turkey escalope

Cupboard

Anchovy fillets

Black pepper

Capers

Cayenne pepper

Cocoa powder, unsweetened

Coconut flour

Coconut milk, tinned

Curry powder

Dijon Mustard

Mustard

Mustard powder

Oil (olive or coconut)

Paprika

Pine nuts

Psyllium husk powder

Sunflower seeds

Tahini

Tomatoes, tinned

Tumeric

Vanilla extract

Walnuts

	Breakfast 130 cal	Lunch 260 cal
Mon	Fruity yoghurt p.179	Salmon with celeriac and kale salad p.194
Tue	Bacon and avocado salad p.181	Salad niçoise p.196
Wed	Scrambled egg whites and smoked salmon p.182	Chicken with Mediterranean vegetables p.198
Thu	Mushroom with tomato and feta p.184	King prawn stuffed pumpkin p.200
Fri	Devilled chicken livers p.185	Baked eggs with anchovies p.189
Sat	Cauliflower fritters p.186	Calamari and crisps p.199
Sun	Scrambled egg and avocado p.183	Kedgeree p.204

Snacks / Sides 60 cal	Dinner 260 cal
Spiced cocoa shot p.221	Aubergine and parma ham salad p.209
Veggies and blue cheese dip p.219	Chicken 'satay' with kale crisps p.212
Berry 'smoothie' p.220	Broccoli and bacon cheese p.214
Coleslaw with sunflower seeds p.218	Pork medallion with mustard and crème fraîche p.211
Cucumber with minted yoghurt dip p.222	Tahini stuffed peppers p.207
Walnuts 10g p.222	Baked haddock with cabbage and courgette p.206
Spiced cocoa shot p.221	Crab cakes and green salad p.216

Week 4 – Shopping List

Fruit and Vegetables

Asparagus
Aubergines
Avocados
Basil
Broccoli
Cauliflower
Celeriac
Celery
Cherry tomatoes
Coriander, fresh
Courgettes
Cucumber
Fennel
Garlic, bulb
Green beans
Kale
Lemons

Mint
Mixed salad leaves
Mushrooms
Peppers, green and red
Portabello mushrooms
Pumpkin (or crown/prince
  squash)
Radishes
Raspberries (or blueberries)
Red cabbage
Red onions
Spinach
Spring greens
Spring onions
Tomatoes
White cabbage

Dairy

Blue cheese
Butter
Cheddar
Crème fraîche
Eggs, large (about 14)

Feta
Parmesan
Ricotta
Yoghurt, natural full fat

Meat and fish

Back bacon

Calamari, fresh

Chicken breast fillets,
  skinless

Chicken livers

Crab meat, fresh or tinned

Haddock fillet

King prawns

Parma ham (or Serrano)

Pork medallions

Salmon fillet

Smoked salmon

Cupboard

Anchovy fillets

Black olives

Black pepper

Capers

Cayenne pepper

Chinese five spice

Cinnamon (sticks
  or powder)

Cocoa powder, unsweetened

Curry powder

Hazelnuts

Mayonnaise

Mustard

Mustard powder

Oil (olive or coconut)

Paprika

Peanut butter
  (100% peanut)

Pecans

Pine nuts

Psyllium husk powder

Salt

Soy sauce

Sunflower seeds

Tahini

Tuna, tinned in springwater

Turmeric

Vanilla extract

Walnuts

THE MEALS

Breakfasts
(130 calories)

Fruity yoghurt

80g full fat natual yoghurt
50g raspberries or 90g blueberries
5g toasted hazelnuts

Prep: 1 min
Washing up: none

Simple! Stir the berries and nuts into the yoghurt. if you buy pre-toasted and chopped hazelnuts, all you need to do here is measure out and combine the ingredients.

Coconut porridge

1 tsp (7g) butter
15ml tinned coconut milk, full fat
15g coconut flour
75ml water
½-1 tsp vanilla extract or pinch of cinnamon

Prep: 5 mins
Washing up: small saucepan, wooden spoon

Slowly heat the butter and coconut milk in a saucepan. Add the coconut flour and water and heat through to a consistency you like. Add the vanilla extract or cinnamon.

Tip: For an optional fibre supplement in your porridge, add a pinch of psyllium husk powder. It is a great bulking agent and readily available from health food shops, but you have to be careful to mix it in well.

Note: Once you are through the low-calorie phase of your plan you can adapt this recipe to include more fat – try doubling the butter quantity, replacing some of the water with coconut milk or adding a beaten egg. As a low-carb porridge alternative it will keep you going for most of the day.

———————————

Bacon and avocado salad

10g bacon
25g avocado
30g mixed salad leaves
9g pine nuts

Prep: 10 mins
Washing up: grill pan, tongs/fork for turning bacon

Heat the grill to medium to high and grill the bacon for 5 minutes on each side. Slice the avocado and place it on a plate with the salad leaves and pine nuts. Add the bacon once cooked. If you prefer your pine nuts toasted, put them in a small heat-proof dish under the grill until lightly browned – but don't leave them too long as they burn quickly.

Scrambled egg whites and smoked salmon

70g smoked salmon
30g mixed salad leaves
30g cherry tomatoes
Dash of oil (ideally olive or coconut)
Whites of 2 large eggs

Prep: 5 mins
Washing up: small non-stick pan, mug, fork and
wooden spoon

Put the salmon, salad and tomatoes (halved if you prefer) onto a plate. Smear the oil around a pan with a piece of paper towel, or use a squirt of spray oil. Heat the pan on the hob. Separate the eggs and put the yolks to one side (you can use them later for mayonnaise or thickening sauces). Lightly whisk the whites in a mug with a fork and pour them into the pan. Stir them as they cook – they will take less than a minute. Remove the pan from the heat and add the scrambled whites to your plate.

Scrambled egg and avocado

30g avocado
30g baby spinach leaves, raw
30g cherry tomatoes
1 large egg

Prep: 7 mins
Washing up: small non-stick pan, mug, fork and
  wooden spoon

Slice the avocado and put it on a plate with the spinach leaves and tomatoes. Warm a pan on the hob and either crack the egg straight in and beat it while it is cooking, or beat it in a mug first. Stir as it cooks and season with some black pepper. Remove it from the heat when done and add the cooked egg to your plate.

Mushroom with tomato and feta

2 large portabello mushrooms
2 medium tomatoes
20g feta

Prep: 7 mins
Washing up: grill pan

Destalk the mushrooms and place them under a hot grill, underside down. Roughly chop the tomato and feta (on your serving plate if you want to save washing up). When the mushrooms start to brown, turn them over. Put the tomato and feta on top, along with a grind of black pepper, and continue to toast the ingredients to your liking.

Devilled chicken livers

40g chicken livers
Pinch of mustard powder or chilli powder
Dash of olive oil
1 medium tomato
20g celery
10g baby leaf spinach
30g avocado

Prep: 15 mins
Washing up: small non-stick pan, spatula

Roughly chop the chicken livers and sprinkle them with mustard / chilli powder. Heat the oil in a pan and seal over a high heat, stirring intermittently. Reduce the heat and continue to stir the livers in the pan until they are cooked through. Roughly chop the tomato and celery and add them to the pan. You can add any herbs (rosemary and thyme work well) if you have them. Add the spinach for the last couple of minutes and cook until wilted. Serve with sliced avocado.

Cauliflower fritters

White of 1 egg
80g cauliflower
30g spring onion
5g butter
12g cheddar, grated

Prep: 15 mins
Washing up: non-stick pan, mixing bowl, grater,
  whisk, spatula

Separate the egg and put the yolk to one side (for use in another recipe). Whisk the white in a bowl until foaming. Grate or finely shred the cauliflower and fold it into the whisked egg white. Finely chop the spring onion and add to the mixture. Leave to sit for a couple of minutes.

Put a pan on to a medium heat and add the butter. Season the cauliflower mixture and pour it slowly into the pan to form individual patties (smaller fritters are easier to flip). Once they start to brown on the underside (after 2-3 minutes) flip them and cook them on the other. Add the grated cheese so that it melts on top.

Note: You can sprinkle over the grated cheddar before flipping if you prefer your cheese toasted.

Poached egg and parma ham

1 tbsp white vinegar
1 large egg
1 slice parma ham
30g mixed salad leaves
5 cherry tomatoes

Prep: 7 mins
Washing up: saucepan, slotted spoon

Boil some water in a pan and add the vinegar. Crack the egg into the centre and poach it for 3 to 4 minutes. In the meantime, put the other ingredients on a plate. When the egg is cooked, add it to the dish.

Tip: If you need a packed lunch option, you can hard-boil the egg instead of poaching it.

Blueberry 'pancake'

White of 1 egg
1 egg, including yolk
Dash of vanilla extract (optional)
Dash of oil (ideally olive or coconut)
45g blueberries

Prep: 10 mins
Washing up: whisk, bowl, spatula and a non-stick
frying pan

Separate the eggs, keeping one yolk for this recipe and putting the other to one side for use in another. Start heating a frying pan over a medium heat. While it is warming up, whisk the egg whites in a bowl until they are roughly the same consistency as whipped cream. Add the single yolk and vanilla extract and whisk it together. Smear the oil around the frying pan with a piece of paper towel (careful: it will be hot). Pour the whisked eggs into the pan to form a single patty. As the underside of the pancake begins to turn golden (about 2-3 minutes) sprinkle the blueberries on top before carefully flipping it over. Remove the pan from the hob and let the residual heat cook the pancake through while you prep your plate.

Lunches

(260 calories)

Baked eggs with anchovies

1 green pepper
2 large eggs
20g anchovy fillets
100g courgette
150g raw spinach

Prep: 20 mins
Washing up: roasting pan

Preheat the oven to 180°C. Halve and deseed the pepper and put it into a roasting pan. Break an egg into each half. Finely chop the anchovy fillets and sprinkle them on top. Slice the courgette and arrange it around the peppers in the roasting pan. Bake for about 10-15 minutes. Towards the end of the cooking time add the spinach to the pan, cover it with foil and return it to the oven for the last few minutes.

Note: If you're not a fan of anchovies – Geoff wasn't – you could replace them with 10g grated cheddar.

Steak and (sort of) chips

50g celeriac
1 tsp olive oil
100g red cabbage
50g green beans
1 tsp butter
60g beef escalope
1 tsp (8g) wholegrain mustard

Prep: 35 mins
Washing up: roasting pan, frying pan, food processor
(optional), tongs/fork for turning steak

Preheat the oven to 180°C. Peel the celeriac and chop into thin slices (you can use the mandolin blade on a food processor, if you have one). Put the slices in the roasting pan, sprinkle them with the oil and bake for about 15-20 minutes until they start to go crisp.

Shred the red cabbage, or chop very finely. When the celeriac is cooked, tip it onto a plate and replace it in the roasting pan with the cabbage and green beans. Cover the pan with foil and return to the oven so the contents can steam until cooked to your liking.

Heat a frying pan until it is really hot, add the butter and sear the steak escalope. Season with some black pepper. Turn the steak to sear the other side, and turn the heat down to cook it through to your taste. Serve it with mustard, the steamed veg and celeriac crisps.

Note: You can peel a whole celeriac and put what you don't use in the fridge for another meal.

Baked mackerel with cauliflower rice

100g cauliflower
3g butter
60g mackerel fillet
Lemon juice (optional)
100g spring greens
100g asparagus
1 tsp olive oil
1 medium tomato
10g feta
Couple of basil leaves

Prep: 30 mins
Washing up: saucepan, roasting pan, wooden spoon,
   food processor or rolling pin/potato masher

Preheat the oven to 180°C. Smash the cauliflower florets in a food processor until fine, or break them up with a rolling pin or potato masher. Add the butter and a small amount of water to a pan and gently cook the cauliflower 'rice' over a medium heat for about 3-5 minutes. Remove it from the heat and allow it to cool.

Season the mackerel and squeeze over some lemon juice. Put it in a roasting pan and bake for around 15 minutes. Chop the spring greens (if not pre-chopped) and, when the mackerel is about halfway through cooking, add them to the roasting pan along with the asparagus. It works best if you reposition the mackerel so it is on top of the veg, as this stops the greens from singeing. Drizzle over the olive oil before returning the fish to the oven.

While it is cooking, chop the tomato and feta and shred the basil. Add these to the cooled cauliflower. You can squeeze over some lemon juice and some black pepper. Serve everything together on a plate.

Tip: You could add curry powder or paprika to the fish seasoning if you feel it needs a bit of livening up.

Note: Once you have finished the restricted calorie phase of your diet you can move on to the more conventional preparation of cauliflower rice: lightly sautéing it in some butter, ghee or a mixture of butter and olive or coconut oil.

Salmon with celeriac and kale salad

85g celeriac
1 tsp olive oil
70g kale, raw
30g radishes, raw
60g salmon fillet
Squeeze of lemon
5g toasted pecans, crushed

Prep: 35 mins
Washing up: roasting pan, food processor (optional)

Preheat the oven to 180°C. Chop the celeriac into 1-inch cubes. Place them in a roasting pan, sprinkle with the oil and cook in the oven for around 25 minutes.

Meanwhile, finely chop the kale and thinly slice the radishes (either with a knife, a potato peeler, or a food processor with a mandolin attachment).

Roughly 10 minutes into the celeriac cooking time, add the salmon to the roasting pan, skin side up. You can squeeze over some lemon juice and a sprinkling of black pepper. The salmon will take about 15 minutes to cook. In the last few minutes, add the pecans to the roasting pan to toast them. Combine everything on a plate to serve. You can use some of the cooking juices to dress the kale salad.

Note: You can prepare a whole celeriac with this method and simply put the cooked chunks you don't use in the fridge for another meal.

Salad niçoise

50g red pepper
1 large egg
30g green beans
1 medium tomato
1 tin (80g) tuna in springwater
30g mixed salad leaves
1 tsp (8g) capers
6 (15g) black olives
8g anchovy fillet
1 tsp mayonnaise
Squeeze of lemon juice

Prep: 18 mins
Washing up: small saucepan, grill pan

Preheat the grill to high and grill the red pepper in two halves, around 5 minutes on each side, until lightly browned. Meanwhile, bring a saucepan of water to the boil and boil the egg for about 6 minutes so that it is still slightly soft in the centre. Run cold water over the egg to stop it cooking further and leave it to cool.

Rinse the pan, add water again and boil the green beans until just softened, about 5 minutes. Drain the beans and refresh them under cold water.

Slice the grilled pepper and the tomato. Pile up all the ingredients on your plate. Add the mayonnaise and lemon juice.

Note: If you prefer, you can simply add the red pepper to the salad raw.

To make your own mayonnaise: Put an egg yolk in a bowl (it is important that the egg is at room temperature, not fridge-cold), add a teaspoon of Dijon mustard and whisk. You can just use a fork, although a hand whisk will work better. While whisking, trickle in about 100-120ml of sunflower oil very slowly. Once the mixture is quite thick, add a tablespoon of white wine vinegar. Season to taste – and you're done!

It will only take around 3-4 minutes to make up your mayonnaise, and you can use up any spare egg yolks from breakfast. The mayo will keep in the fridge if sealed for a couple of days – but remember that a teaspoon will contain 30 calories.

Chicken with Mediterranean vegetables

100g aubergine
90g courgette
75g green pepper
75g skinless chicken breast
1 tsp olive oil
25g mixed salad leaves
Couple of basil leaves, shredded
6 (15g) black olives
5g feta

Prep: 25 mins
Washing up: grill pan

Cut the aubergine, courgette, pepper and chicken into thin strips and mix them together in a grill pan. Brush it all with the olive oil and season with black pepper. Bake under a medium to hot grill for 15 minutes – turning half-way through cooking time – or until the chicken is cooked through. Take care with the chicken as it can dry out easily. Mix up the salad leaves, basil, olives and feta on a plate and place the grilled chicken and vegetables on top.

Calamari and crisps

80g celeriac
120g spring greens
60g cherry tomatoes
50g green beans
Dash of oil (ideally olive or coconut)
170g fresh calamari
½ tsp paprika

Prep: 30 mins
Washing up: roasting pan, frying pan, spatula,
food processor (optional)

Preheat the oven to 180°C. Chop the celeriac into thin slices (you can use the mandolin blade on a food processor, if you have one) and tip them into a roasting pan. Cook in the oven for about 20 minutes until the celeriac is crispy. Push it to one side in the roasting pan and add the spring greens (sliced), tomatoes and green beans and cook for a further 5 minutes. While this is cooking, heat up the frying pan and spray/ smear it with oil. Fry the calamari with a sprinkling of paprika for a couple of minutes until opaque and cooked through. Serve it tossed on the veg with the celeriac crisps on top.

King prawn stuffed pumpkin

200g pumpkin
1tsp olive oil
140g king prawns
Sprinkle of paprika
1 medium tomato
60g courgette
100g mushrooms
7g pine nuts
Handful of fresh coriander, roughly chopped

Prep: 35 mins
Washing up: roasting pan, saucepan,
*   spatula/wooden spoon*

Preheat the oven to 180°C. Cut a wide wedge from the pumpkin (about 200g, seeds removed). You can save the rest of the pumpkin for another dish if you're not cooking this recipe in bulk. Brush the pumpkin wedge with the olive oil and place it skin-down in a roasting tray. Bake in the oven for about 30 minutes.

After about 20 minutes, spoon some of the cooking juices from the pumpkin roasting tray into a saucepan and use it to sear the prawns with a sprinkle of paprika. Continue to fry them until cooked through and pink.

Chop the tomato, courgette and mushrooms and fry them with the prawns for about 5 minutes, until cooked to your liking. Toss in the pine nuts towards the end to toast them a little.

Remove the pumpkin from the oven when cooked and put it on a plate. Tip the prawn and vegetable mixture into the pumpkin wedge cavity. Top with fresh coriander.

Note: Roasted pumpkin tastes amazing when in season but you could use a marrow or another type of squash if pumpkin isn't available.

Aubergine and spinach bake with mozzarella

(serves 2 – 260 calories per serving)

300g aubergine

1 tsp olive oil (plus a bit more for spraying)

2 cloves garlic

Selection of herbs (your choice from rosemary,
basil, oregano and thyme)

400g tinned tomatoes

1 egg

55g ricotta

35g full fat yoghurt

1 tsp mustard

150g green beans

150g spinach

10g parmesan

Prep: 35 mins
Washing up: ovenproof dish, saucepan, fork, mixing
bowl and steaming/boiling pan(s)

Preheat the oven to 180°C. Cut the aubergine into
slices about half a centimetre thick and arrange in an
ovenproof dish. Drizzle with olive oil and bake for
about 20 minutes.

Crush or grate the garlic and cook it in a saucepan with a dash of oil over a medium heat, along with any herbs you are using. Stir until the garlic starts to soften. Add the tinned tomatoes and turn the heat up so that the sauce reduces. Season as required.

While this is reducing, beat an egg in a bowl and mix it with the ricotta, yoghurt and mustard to make a white sauce.

About halfway through the aubergine cooking time put the green beans into a pan of boiling water (or into a steaming pan over boiling water) and simmer (or steam) until cooked to your liking. Drain them and season to serve.

Remove the aubergine from the oven when softened. Add the spinach to the tomato sauce and stir it in until it starts to wilt. Pour the tomato sauce over the aubergines, blob the white sauce on top and then sprinkle with the grated parmesan. Return it to the oven until it is bubbling and golden.

Serve on a plate with the beans on the side.

Kedgeree
(serves 2 – 260 calories per serving)

2 eggs
200g cauliflower
2 anchovy fillets
110g salmon fillets
1 tsp olive oil
8g curry powder
65g spinach
Selection of herbs, such as coriander and chives
Squeeze of lemon juice
40g full fat natual yoghurt

Prep: 20 mins
Washing up: saucepan x 2, spatula/wooden spoon,
  food processor or rolling pin/potato masher

Put the eggs in a pan of boiling water and simmer until they are hardboiled (about 8 minutes). Meanwhile, smash the cauliflower florets in a food processor until fine, or break them up with a rolling pin or potato masher, or simply chop finely. Finely slice the anchovy and cut the salmon fillets into chunks.

Put a second pan on a medium heat, add the olive oil and lightly cook the cauliflower. As the steam builds up (1-2 minutes) add the curry powder, anchovy and salmon. Cook until the salmon starts to turn opaque (about 5 minutes), turning occasionally. Stir in the spinach and let it wilt. Slice the hardboiled eggs and add them to the pan. Season and squeeze over the lemon juice. Serve with a blob of yoghurt.

Suppers

(260 calories)

Baked haddock with cabbage and garlic courgettes

150g courgette
2 cloves garlic
1 tsp olive oil
125g red cabbage
100g asparagus
125g haddock fillet
1 tbsp capers
Squeeze of lemon juice

Prep: 35 mins
Washing up: roasting pan and food
  processor (optional)

Preheat the oven to 180°C. Roughly chop the courgette and put it in a roasting pan with the garlic and a drizzle of olive oil. Bake in the oven for 15 minutes. Meanwhile, finely chop the cabbage (or shred using the mandolin blade of the food processor).

When the courgette has been in the oven for about 15 minutes remove it temporarily from the pan and put to one side. Put the cabbage and asparagus in the pan and place the haddock fillet on top. Sprinkle over the capers and add a squeeze of lemon juice. Put the courgettes back in, on top of the fish and veg, and roast it all for another 15 minutes or until the haddock is cooked through.

Tahini stuffed peppers

100g courgette
1 tbsp tahini
45g ricotta
Juice of half a lemon
1 green pepper, halved and deseeded
30g avocado
30g mixed salad leaves

Prep: 35 mins
Washing up: mixing bowl, wooden spoon,
   roasting pan

Preheat the oven to 180°C. Finely chop the courgette and mix it in a bowl with the tahini, ricotta and lemon juice. Add a few turns of black pepper. Place the halves of green pepper in a roasting dish and spoon the mixture into the cavities. Roast them in the oven for about 30 minutes. Slice the avocado and serve with the salad leaves and cooked peppers.

Turkey escalope with mushrooms

50g celeriac
1 tsp olive oil (plus a bit more for spraying)
65g green beans
85g spinach
95g mushrooms
85g turkey escalope
1 tsp Dijon mustard
15g crème fraîche

Prep: 30 mins
Washing up: frying pan, roasting pan, spatula, food processor (optional)

Preheat the oven to 180°C. Peel the celeriac and chop it into thin slices (you can use the mandolin blade on a food processor, if you have one). Spray it with oil and cook in the oven for about 20 minutes, until crispy. Once done, place it on a plate and replace it in the roasting pan with the green beans and spinach. Cover the pan with foil and return to the oven so the contents can steam until cooked to your liking.

Meanwhile, slice the mushrooms and put them in a hot frying pan with the oil and the turkey escalope. Fry the escalope for about 3 minutes on each side, or until cooked through, then put it on a plate to rest. Add the mustard and crème fraîche to the pan and mix it through. Add some black pepper then pour the frying pan contents over the turkey. Serve with the vegetables.

Aubergine and parma ham salad

150g aubergine
50g fennel
2 tsp olive oil
10g pine nuts
30g mixed salad leaves
55g cherry tomatoes
1 slice Parma ham

Prep: 15 mins
Washing up: grill pan

Heat the grill to moderate. Cut the aubergine into strips and the fennel into thin wedges and drizzle with the oil. Grill for about 10 minutes, turning halfway through cooking time, until browned. Add the pine nuts to the grill pan at the last minute – but watch that they don't burn. Serve with salad leaves, chopped cherry tomatoes and the Parma ham.

Courgette pizzas with salmon fillet

100g courgette
1 tsp olive oil
60g salmon fillet
50g green or yellow pepper
1 medium tomato
20g mozzarella
8g anchovy fillets
Couple of basil leaves

Prep: 20 mins
Washing up: grill pan

Heat the grill to moderate to high. Chop the courgette in half lengthways, drizzle with the olive oil and place it in a grill pan. Cook under the grill (initially cut-side down) with the salmon fillet (skin-side up). Grill them for 12-16 minutes, turning both halfway through cooking. Meanwhile, roughly chop the pepper, tomato, mozzarella, anchovy fillets and basil leaves. Place these on the courgette once it is turned over and continue to cook everything until golden.

Pork medallion with mustard and crème fraîche sauce

85g red onion
1 tsp olive oil
65g pork medallions
120g broccoli
2 tsp wholegrain mustard
15g crème fraîche

Prep: 20 mins
Washing up: frying pan, steaming/boiling pan(s),
*   spatula*

Chop the onion into wedges and fry it in the olive oil over a moderate heat. When the onion has softened, add the pork medallions to the pan and continue to fry for another 7-10 minutes or until the meat is cooked through. Meanwhile, break the broccoli into florets and add to a saucepan of boiling water (or into a steam pan over boiling water) and simmer (or steam) for 5-10 minutes until just softened. Mix the wholegrain mustard and crème fraîche in the frying pan, and serve.

Chicken 'satay' with kale crisps

60g chicken breast fillets

Chinese five spice

2 tsp soy sauce

10g peanut butter (100% peanuts)

1 tsp vinegar (or water)

100g kale, shredded

1 tsp olive oil

75g cucumber

Prep: 20 mins

Washing up: grill pan, bowl and mixing spoon, tongs

Heat the grill to moderate to high. Cut the chicken into strips and mix it in a bowl with the Chinese five spice and one teaspoon of the soy sauce. Place under the grill for 8-10 minutes, turning occasionally, until cooked through. Mix the peanut butter with the other teaspoon of soy and with a teaspoon of vinegar.

Place the cooked chicken on a plate and top it with the sauce. Put the shredded kale into the grill pan and drizzle with the oil. Grill the kale on a medium heat for a few minutes. Watch it carefully and turn it over a couple of times – once it is done it will have the texture of crispy seaweed. Cut the cucumber into strips and serve the veg with the 'satay' chicken.

Poached eggs and mushrooms

100g green beans
2 portabello mushrooms
2 tsp white vinegar
2 large eggs
13g cheddar

Prep: 15 mins
Washing up: steaming/boiling pan(s), grill pan,
*   cheese grater, slotted spoon*

Put the green beans into a pan of boiling water (or
into a steam pan over boiling water) and simmer (or
steam) for 5-10 minutes until softened to your liking.
Heat the grill to moderate to high. Destalk the mushrooms and grill them for 5 minutes on each side.

Meanwhile, drain the beans, refresh them under
cold water and place them on a plate. Rinse the pan
and use it to bring more water to the boil. Swirl in the
vinegar and then crack the eggs into the centre of the
pan and poach them for about 3 minutes. Lift them
out (ideally with a slotted spoon) when they are loosely
formed but not completely cooked. Turn the mushrooms underside up and place the eggs on top. Grate
the cheese over the top and grill the stack to finish off
the cooking and toast the cheese. Serve with the beans.

Broccoli and bacon cheese

(serves 2 – 260 calories per serving)

30g back bacon
1 tsp olive oil
150g broccoli
130g ricotta cheese
1 tbsp crème fraîche
8g mustard
1 egg yolk
20g parmesan, grated

Prep: 20 mins
Washing up: saucepan with lid, ovenproof
dish, whisk, slotted spoon

Heat the grill to moderate. Slice the bacon and put it in a saucepan with the olive oil. Fry until crispy (7-10 minutes). Transfer the bacon to an ovenproof dish.

Carefully wipe the fat from the pan with some kitchen towel (caution: it will be hot) to avoid the juices spitting when it is next on the heat. Roughly chop or break up the broccoli and add it to the pan with some water. Cover with a lid and steam for about 3-4 minutes.

When it is just tender but still bright green, transfer the broccoli to the ovenproof dish with the bacon.

Drain the pan and tip in the ricotta, crème fraîche and mustard. Mix and season well. Warm the sauce through until it starts to bubble gently. Remove it from the heat and whisk in the egg yolk, before putting back on the heat briefly to thicken up to your liking. Pour the sauce over the broccoli and bacon. Sprinkle it with grated parmesan and place it under the grill until golden.

Crab cakes and green salad
(serves 2 – 260 calories per serving)

For the crab cakes:
50g spinach
4 eggs
25g crème fraîche
2 anchovy fillets
Handful of coriander
75g crab meat, either fresh, dressed or tinned

For the salad:
50g cucumber
30g mixed salad leaves
1 tsp olive oil (or walnut oil, if you prefer)
Squeeze of lemon juice

Prep: 20 mins
Washing up: muffin tray, frying pan, mixing
*   bowl and fork*

Preheat the oven to 180°C and lightly grease a muffin tray with a small amount of butter. Wilt the spinach in a frying pan for a minute or two. Remove it from the heat, squeeze out any excess water and allow it to cool. Beat the eggs in a bowl with the crème fraîche. Chop the anchovy fillets and coriander and add them to the egg mix. Stir in the crab and spinach and pour the mixture into the cups in the muffin tray. Bake for about 10 minutes until set.

Slice the cucumber and place it on a plate with the salad leaves. Dress with the oil and a squeeze of lemon and serve with the cooked crab cakes.

Snacks / Sides

(60 calories)

Coleslaw with sunflower seeds

(makes 3 portions – 60 caloties per portion)

60g red cabbage

60g white cabbage

50g full fat natural yoghurt

1 round tsp crème fraîche

12g sunflower seeds

Prep: 5 mins

*Washing up: mixing bowl and spoon, grater or
food processor*

Shred the cabbage with a grater or food processor and
mix it in a bowl with the yoghurt, crème fraîche and
sunflower seeds. Season to taste. Split the coleslaw into
three portions and keep the extras for another day.

Veggies and blue cheese dip

50g celery or cucumber
1 flat tsp mayonnaise
2 tsp water
10g blue cheese

Prep: 3 mins
Washing up: small bowl or cup and a fork
  for mixing

Cut the celery or cucumber into batons. Mix the mayonnaise with the water and blue cheese in a bowl. Add a little black pepper, and get dunking.

Note: If you want to make your own mayonnaise it is very simple. You can find the recipe on p.197

Berry 'smoothie'

50g raspberries or 45g blueberries, fresh or frozen
1 tbsp full fat yoghurt
1 tsp psyllium husk powder
200-300ml cold water

Prep: 4 mins
Washing up: mini blender (ideally)

Place all the ingredients in the blender and pulse until smooth.

Note: Psyllium husk powder is a great bulking agent and an excellent source of fibre. It is readily available from health food shops but it needs to be thoroughly mixed in.

Tip: It is hard to get a decent consistency for this smoothie without a blender, especially if you are using frozen berries. A mini blender is often a worthwhile investment: it won't take up much room in your cupboard and you can pick up a powerful one for under £30. I use mine every day for small-portion blending and mixing.

Spiced cocoa shot

7g unsweetened cocoa powder
5g unsalted butter
150-200ml boiling water

Possible infusions to add:
Cinnamon stick, chunk of peeled root ginger, strip of
    vanilla pod, star anise, 2-4 whole cloves or a thick
    slice of orange peel

Prep: 2 mins
Washing up: bowl and whisk, or a mini blender

Mix together the ingredients in a bowl with a whisk,
or in a mini blender. Pour into a mug and add the
infusion of your choice.

Note: You can use powdered spices instead of the infusions, but their flavours tend to be stronger so go easy.

Cucumber with minted yoghurt dip

100g cucumber
2 tsp fresh mint
50g full fat Greek yoghurt

Prep: 5 mins
Washing up: bowl and spoon for mixing

Cut the cucumber into batons. Roughly chop the mint so that it is quite fine and a little bruised and mix it with the yoghurt in a bowl. Season to taste. Get dipping!

Nuts

Nuts are amazingly nutritious but their calorie content can add up fast. A snack portion for these purposes is roughly 10g (a fair handful), which really isn't much, but they are a great source of protein and will keep you going longer than you think.

Snack hack – slow boiled broth

This is certainly not one for vegetarians but it is astoundingly nutritious, low-calorie and satiating.

- 1-2kg raw bones (chicken, beef or lamb)
- 2 handfuls of veg (onions, leeks, carrots)
- Small handful of herbs (rosemary, thyme, bay leaves)
- Splash of cider vinegar, or lemon juice

Put the bones, including all the gristly cartilage, into a large pan – a slow cooker or an ovenproof pot with a lid. Add the veg and herbs. Cover with water and season with some black pepper.

If you are using a slow cooker, leave it bubbling away for about three days but do check the water level intermittently. To oven-cook, put the lid on the pot and leave it simmering on low (70-100°C) overnight.

Once the broth has been drained and cooled you can freeze it in portion sizes and heat it up when needed. As an emergency snack, a cup of this with a good squeeze of lemon and a sprinkling of salt is both warming and fortifying. It is full of minerals that can be hard to access – especially on a calorie-restricted diet – and does the same job in one cup as loads of expensive dietary supplements. You can also use it as a base for soups and sauces. It will really make you glow.

Jen Whitington is a fitness trainer and co-producer of the *Fixing Dad* film. As wife of Anthony Whitington, she was instrumental in devising and seeing through Geoff's diet and fitness plan.

For additional information and support go to fixingdad.com